Basic readings in
Medical Sociology

Basic readings in Medical Sociology

edited by DAVID TUCKETT
& JOSEPH M. KAUFERT

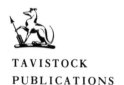

TAVISTOCK
PUBLICATIONS

First published in 1978
by Tavistock Publications Limited
11 *New Fetter Lane, London* EC4P 4EE

ISBN 0 422 76280 6 (*hardback*)
ISBN 0 422 76290 3 (*paperback*)

© *David Tuckett and Joseph M. Kaufert*
Filmset by Northumberland Press Ltd.
and printed in Great Britain by
Cambridge University Press

Contents

Acknowledgements

The readings in this book have previously been published in other places. The following individuals and bodies are thanked for permission to reprint.

Reading 1: Plenum Publishing Corporation for 'The Measurement of Family Activities and Relationships' by George Brown and Michael Rutter, *Human Relations* (1966) **19**:241–63. **Reading 2**: Cambridge University Press for 'The Measurement of Expressed Emotion in the Families of Psychiatric Patients' by Christine Vaughn and Julian Leff, *British Journal of Social and Clinical Psychology* (1976) **15**:157–65. **Reading 3**: The *Millbank Memorial Fund Quarterly* for 'An Appraisal with Implications for Theoretical Development of Some Epidemiological Work on Heart Disease' by Edward A. Suchman (1967) **XLV** (2) part 2:109–13. **Reading 4**: The American Sociological Association for Tables 1–4 from 'Parental Interest and Children's Self-conceptions' by Morris Rosenberg, *Sociometry* **26**:35–49, March. **Reading 5**: The *University of London Bulletin* for 'Does Medicine Need Sociology?' by Margot Jefferys,

(1974) No. 6:7–9, March. **Reading 6**: The *Lancet* for 'History-taking for Medical Students: Deficiencies in Performance' by G. Peter Maguire and Derek Rutter, (1976) ii:556–58, September 11. **Reading 7**: The *Journal of Social Issues* for 'The Psychological Meaning of Mental Illness in the Family' by Marian Radke-Yarrow, Charlotte Green Schwartz, Harriet S. Murphy, and Leila Calhoun Deasy, (1955) 11(4):12–24. **Reading 8**: The *British Journal of Psychiatry* for 'The Influence of Family Life on the Course of Schizophrenic Disorders' by George W. Brown, J. L. T. Birley, and John K. Wing (1972), 121:248–58. **Reading 9**: The American Academy of Pediatrics for 'Behavioral Observations on Parents Anticipating the Death of a Child' by Stanford Barton Friedman, Paul Chodoff, John W. Mason, and David A. Hamburg, *Pediatrics* (1963) 32:610–25. **Reading 10**: The *Sociological Review* for 'Social Class Variations in Health Care and in the Nature of General Practice Consultations' by Ann Cartwright and Maureen O'Brien, in M. Stacey (ed.), *The Sociology of the National Health Service, Sociological Review Monograph No. 22*. **Reading 11**: The Family Service Association of America for 'Clash in Perspective between Worker and Client' by John E. Mayer and Noel Timms, *Social Casework* (1969) 50:32–40, January. **Reading 12**: The London Borough of Southwark for 'The Mobile Health Clinic: A Report on the First Year's Work' by Joseph E. Epsom, Mimeo (1969). **Reading 13**: Oxford Journals, Oxford University Press for 'Factors Influencing the Demand for Primary Medical Care in Women Aged 20–44 Years: A Preliminary Report' by Michael Banks, S. A. A. Beresford, D. C. Morrell, J. J. Waller, and C. J. Watkins, *International Journal of Epidemiology* (1975)4(3):189–95. **Reading 14**: Pergamon Press Ltd. for 'Pathways to the Doctor – From Person to Patient' by Irving Kenneth Zola, *Social Science and Medicine* (1973) 7:677–89. **Reading 15**: Pitman Medical Publishing Co., Ltd. for an extract from *The Doctor, His Patient and the Illness* by Michael Balint, Pitman Medical Company Ltd, London, 2nd Edition 1964. **Reading 16**: Routledge & Kegan Paul for an extract from *Going to See the Doctor* by Gerry Stimson and Barbara Webb, 1975, London. **Reading 17**: The University of Chicago Press for 'Uncertainty in Medical Prognosis' by Fred Davis, *American Journal of Sociology* (1960) 66:41–47. **Reading 18**: Pergamon Press Ltd. for 'Vocabularies of Realism in Professional Socialization' by Joan Stelling and Rue Bucher, *Social Science and Medicine* (1973) 7:661–75. **Reading 19**: Professor A. Querido for 'Forecast and Follow-up' from the *British Journal of Social and Preventive Medicine* (1959) 13:33–49. **Reading 20**: *The New England Journal of Medicine* for 'Reduction of Post–Operative Pain by Encouragement and Instruction of Patients' by Lawrence D. Egbert, George E. Battit,

Claude E. Welch, and Marshall K. Bartlett, (1964) **270**:825–27. **Reading 21**: The American Sociological Association for 'Children, Stress, and Hospitalization' by James K. Skipper and Robert C. Leonard, *Journal of Health and Social Behavior* (1968) **9**:275–87. **Reading 22**: Macmillan Publishing Co., Inc. for 'The Sociology of Time and Space in an Obstetrical Hospital' by William R. Rosengren and Spencer DeVault, in Eliot Friedson (ed.), *The Hospital in Modern Society*, 1964, New York. **Reading 23**: Cambridge University Press for an extract from *Institutionalism and Schizophrenia* by John K. Wing and George W. Brown, 1970, Cambridge. **Reading 24**: Macmillan Publishing Co., Inc. for 'Alienation and the Social Structure' by Rose Laub Coser, in Eliot Friedson (ed.), *The Hospital in Modern Society*, 1964, New York. **Reading 25**: The Bethlem Royal Hospital and the Maudsley Hospital for 'Depression: A Sociological View' by George W. Brown, *Maudsley Gazette* (1976), Summer. **Reading 26**: The American Medical Association for 'Coronary Heart Disease in the Western Collaborative Group Study: Final Follow-up Experience of Eight and One-half Years' by Ray H. Rosenman, Richard J. Brand, C. David Jenkins, Meyer Friedman, Reuben Straus, and Moses Wurm, the *American Medical Association Journal* (1975) **233**:872–77, Copyright 1975, American Medical Association. **Reading 27**: Reprinted from *Behavioral Science*, Volume 8, No. 1. 1963, by permission of James G. Miller, M.D., Ph.D., Editor. **Reading 28**: The *Sociological Review* for 'Medicine as an Institution of Social Control' by Irving Kenneth Zola, (1972) **20**:487–504. **Reading 29**: Marion Boyars Publishers Ltd. for 'Medical Nemesis' by Ivan Illich, the *Lancet* (1974) i:918–21, May 11. **Reading 30**: The *Lancet* for 'Health – A Demystification of Medical Technology' by Halfdan Mahler, ii:829–33, November, 1975.

Editors' introduction

This volume is intended as a companion to *An Introduction to Medical Sociology* (Tuckett 1976) and is an attempt to bring together in an economical and manageable way many of the source materials discussed in it. A small book of articles is necessarily selective. Our aim, therefore, has been to choose work which provides someone coming to the field with the chance to assess the direction, quality, scope, and utility of the subject. Since there were bound to be omissions, we have concentrated on contributions which are otherwise difficult to obtain and which complement *An Introduction to Medical Sociology*. For these latter reasons several important works are missing. Nonetheless we hope that this reader will prove useful to the full range of workers in the health and social services and to those in medical sociology.

We had two additional considerations in mind when selecting the individual readings. First, we wanted to include those contributions which reflect some of the more interesting ways in which medical sociologists look at particular aspects of medicine, health, or disease.

Second, we attempted to select papers which not only convey an interesting perspective on a topic but also make a systematic attempt to test the validity of ideas. We particularly emphasize validity and therefore methodological considerations because it is in this respect as well as for ideas and insights that we believe medical sociology will be judged, and not only by outsiders.

Two aspects to medical sociological work can be distinguished. On the one hand, there has been the attempt to develop knowledge by rethinking various received or standard perspectives on medical issues. The work of Parsons (for example, 1951) and Freidson (for example, 1970), the latter rethinking some of the former's rethinking of medical ideas concerning the nature of the doctor–patient encounter, and of Goffman (1968) on the social-psychological implication of hospital admission, are well-known examples. On the other hand, but not necessarily divorced from work-generating ideas, there has been work directed towards the substantiation of a particular point of view. Many of the papers selected for this volume (for example Readings 23 and 24) illustrate this aspect of work.

Sociological work which has concentrated primarily on the generation of ideas and perspectives has been important. Quite often our main experience in reaction to encountering a medical situation may be to use our data in order to rethink a conventional perspective. It may be this perspective and the more or less developed assumptions which underlie it which we wish to challenge before we do anything else. Its taken-for-granted logical structure and theory may well make us uncomfortable. Some sociologists want to expose the logical weaknesses of existing theory and to develop a new set of theories and assumptions before testing them.

A number of contributions in this book derive their value from the fact that they consist primarily of a formal consideration of medical settings from a hitherto unconsidered point of view. Thus, previous descriptions and explanations may be rethought and earlier sets of assumptions about the nature of social reality or the behaviour of social actors may be reconsidered. Zola's discussion of the factors turning a person into a patient (Reading 14) and Stimson and Webb's consideration of the doctor–patient interaction (Reading 16), are good examples. Both contributions demonstrate how inadequate assumptions about social action have handicapped previous thinking and research.

The ways in which ideas and perspectives about a sociological issue are developed are many and as is commonly argued, there can be no such thing as a unitary methodology for this task. Different people work creatively in different ways and all sorts of serendipitous meetings and chance occurrences can lead to the familiar being perceived in a new way. A number of the most interesting medical sociological ideas have been derived by sociologists who never formally undertook empirical research at all. Yet again ideas have been generated as the result of changing fashions in the way sociologists look at the situations they study. Linked sets of assumptions underlying structural-functional, conflict, symbolic-interactionist, ethnomethodological, and Marxist perspectives have all dominated at different times and each has generated ideas such that we examine medical situations in very different ways as a result.

However, it is in our view at some stage necessary, when considering the achievement of medical sociology as a whole, for workers not only to develop and generate ideas and theories but also to face the equally demanding and creative task of demonstrating that their ideas are ones which have a well-established basis in fact. Such activity is not noticeably widespread among medical sociologists at the present time (see, for example, the recent proceedings of a BSA conference on medical sociology (Dingwall *et al.* 1977)). As a consequence of the failure to test ideas we find that a great deal of medical sociological work, although interesting, is rather unconvincing.

We do not think that the generation of ideas is the only or even the main task of sociologists. Nor do we consider the testing of ideas a job for 'foot-soldiers'. If medical sociologists are to be taken seriously and to justify themselves as undertaking useful activities we need to be able to demonstrate that our ideas do describe and explain the medical world and related issues. It is for this reason that although contributions primarily important for their introduction of new ideas and perspectives are not excluded from the present volume, we have emphasized contributions which submit ideas to test against the facts. It is also for this reason that we have included four papers under the heading of 'Sociology as a science' and in selecting those papers have chosen contributions that set out a particular, so-called positivistic, approach to the testing of ideas. While there may be many ways of developing ideas, we believe there is essentially only one logic for testing them. Also, it will be noted that many of the contributions we have included are drawn from the early stages of the development of medical sociology. In part this reflects the fact that the subject has not been developed in the way it might. Quite often the original work has not been pursued by later investigators.

We have referred to systematic testing against the facts. Now, if there is one thing that almost all sociologists will agree on, it is that what are called facts are frequently shown to be more or less well-disguised assertions based on a particular set of value judgements and so-called domain assumptions. This is often the case and we should never lose sight of it. At the same time we cannot accept that philosophical doubts about the nature of evidence and enquiry can be used, as indeed they are, as an excuse for a kind of nihilistic relativism which rejects the possibility of inter-subjective judgement and thus equates properly conducted empirical enquiry with individual opinions about the social world. It may be difficult to establish facts on which to base understanding but it is utterly foolish to allow that to make us give up the attempt. Difficult and problematic as the logic and practice of social research actually is, it is all that separates sociology from punditry. Although some ideas can be made convincing without reference to empirical work most can be held with any confidence only as the result of properly conducted social enquiry.

We have referred several times to properly conducted social enquiry because we believe that there is a sufficiently developed middle ground in sociology for a broad agreement to be reached as to what is the proper method for testing social theories and one largely independent of the different ideas we are trying to test. It involves a logic and a particular approach to the problems of research design, measurement, and analysis. We sketch its main features only briefly here, and without a detailed explanation of terms, because it has been outlined more fully in *An Introduction to Medical Sociology*.

The logic of research to which we refer is one based on the premise that the best we can do when we draw inferences from our observation of the social world is *to make a case* for the inference. The research worker's audience must be given grounds for believing that alternative interpretations of observable phenomena are less likely to be accurate than his own. That is, the research worker must anticipate such alternative interpretations and then initiate procedures to try to falsify them and so put his readers in a situation where they can make an informed judgement between them. We do not deny that inference will always remain a matter of judgement and argument. It is not possible to prove a theory. But the creative use of methodological procedures and argument, preferably combined in a series of studies, can provide the accumulation of knowledge which can make theories more or less acceptable. The central requirement of this logic, therefore, is that research workers directly face the issue of alternative interpretations and set out their arguments before their audience. Confidence depends on how well the case for a particular interpretation has been made.

Alternative interpretations which contradict a research worker's inference will threaten internal validity or external validity. That is, they suggest either that the study does not show what it purports to or that its results cannot be generalized to the situations to which the research worker claims it can. Alternative interpretations are relevant at each stage of research: that is, of design, measurement, and analysis. Proper design involves such things as the appropriate selection of samples (relevant to external validity), the choice of appropriate comparison groups, the selection of a longitudinal or cross-sectional design (all relevant to internal validity), and so on. In contrast to the latter stages, traditions in regard to research design are so well established in sociology, as well as in other disciplines, that they need not be considered further.

The methodological section of this volume (Sociology as a science) contains two readings which contribute substantially to ideas about measurement. At the heart of this matter one comes back, inevitably, to one issue: how we should interpret observed events (be they situations directly observed, reports, official statistics, answers on a questionnaire or interview, or any other form of observation). Thus, does that facial expression mean a doctor is bored? Does that emotion indicate dissatisfaction? To what does that 'yes' refer? And so on. Whether the data-collection method is a questionnaire, a scheduled interview, a semi-structured interview, participant observation, or any other method, the crucial question remains: has the interpretation of the data been imposed arbitrarily or is there evidence that formal procedures have been used to establish it in such a way that readers can make an informed assessment of its validity *for the purpose*? We have to impose meaning; the question is how to make a case for the particular meaning we impose.

It is a failure to provide the reader with the confidence to believe in the interpretations that are offered (or in some cases the failure to recognize that interpretations are being made at all) which is the central weakness of so much sociological research. For example, in an area of study in which one of us is involved, standard schedule interviews (with fixed questions and fixed choice answers) are used. Thus respondents are asked: 'Were you on the whole very satisfied/satisfied/mixed feelings/rather dissatisfied/dissatisfied with your last visit to the doctor?' Here the difficulty is in knowing to what do the investigators think the respondents refer, and to what do the investigators think the respondents think the investigators refer, were the respondents to answer the question seriously. Do respondents all attach the same meaning to the categories? What aspects of the consultation do they evaluate and from what standpoint? Are respondents making statements about the doctor 'as a person' or as a medical technician, etc? Unless the investigators supply openly the answers to these questions it is hard to see how we can interpret their results. We should make it clear that this is not a universal indictment of the schedule interview. We do not advocate ending the worthwhile attempt to quantify respondents' answers and its replacement solely by in-depth exploration of a few cases and the anecdotal reporting of findings. It is rather a plea for investigators to face the interpretative issues involved in a schedule interview before they embark on using it.

We think the logic of a solution to problems of measurement is available and Reading 1, in which Brown and Rutter discuss their attempts to develop a way of assessing aspects of family life, provides an example of a tradition which is quite well established not only in sociology and social psychiatry but in psychology and ethnology. Their emphasis is on the need for considerable and well-planned developmental work in which different interpretations of data can be thoroughly considered and through which the method's reliability can be formally studied. The rules of interpretation must be made clear, the particular method compared to alternative approaches to data-collection and observers trained so that independently they can reach the same interpretation of the data. Only after this is the reader of a research report in a position to assess the validity of the interpretations that have been made. If the rules are clear then interpretations can be accepted, rejected, or contested more productively.

Reading 2 in which Vaughn and Leff extend the Brown and Rutter family interview method by simplifying it and making it less time-consuming (in a controlled way) is included to show that the approach we are advocating can be made economical. Given proper developmental work there is no reason for only the four-hour interviews used by Brown and Rutter to be necessary to ensure valid data. There is no objection, in principle, to applying the same logic to the valid testing of the most complex sociomedical ideas. Furthermore, the logic of the method is applicable to verbal and non-verbal aspects of an interview, as well as to questionnaires and the different types of observation.

The task of completing adequate analysis of sociological data and then reporting it has always presented problems in social research. Any type of study can present us with difficulties of interpretation because of the way the analysis has been conducted but here we take our example from intensive studies of the doctor–patient relationship. Whereas the schedule interview approach discussed above avoids the problem of selecting data for analysis (sometimes referred to as coding) by providing fixed-choice responses (with all the potential problems of interpretation we have been discussing), research workers using intensive in-depth interviewing face the same problem later. Intensive or qualitative data are usually fascinating and have a direct human quality but provide a mass of data which is difficult to summarize. The most common approach is to present results by selecting examples which illustrate theoretical points. But this in turn raises many questions. How has the material been selected? How many patients do as the doctor says? How many discuss their problem with friends? How important is such discussion to what is done with the doctor's advice? How often does the patient initiate a request? How often does the doctor ignore such requests? When are the explanations advocated by investigators applicable? And so on. With only illustrative examples to go on we cannot know. But in order to be able to evaluate the theories and ideas that are generated from such intensive material, and to relate them to other work and to the accumulation of evidence, it is necessary to answer such questions.

We believe that intensive interview data can be analyzed and reported in a valid way if procedures for systematically defining and recording the occurrence of the phenomena in which we are interested are developed. Thus, to continue with the example above, we can define (in the manner indicated by Brown and Rutter) what constitutes a patient's request and examine the data to see when, how often, and in what circumstances the doctor responds in various ways to the request. We can define discussion with friends, reappraisal and reinterpretation of the doctor's advice and different degrees to which this is done, and then we can examine different ways in which the advice is followed or otherwise. This process of precisely defining variables is best done as part of the original measurement, but it can be done later. Once we have the ideas and insights as to what we want to examine we go on to use our technical ingenuity to find indicators with which to test them. We can then answer how often, in what circumstances, and with what results the different phenomena occur.

If we can develop indicators to categorize our data systematically in terms of the theoretical concepts we have developed, then we can proceed to analyze it more thoroughly and to present it more systematically. Examples can then be systematically sampled and their typicality stated. As Rosenberg's contribution (Reading 4) demonstrates, we can then use powerful techniques to elaborate and test our theories by falsifying rival explanations. In the course of such work new theoretical ideas may occur. Suchman's paper (Reading 3) shows how the analysis itself can lead to much more coherent thinking and to a systematic accumulation of knowledge.

It may come as a surprise to some readers if we say that the kind of techniques we have discussed in the last two paragraphs are unusual in medical sociological work. Yet we find it hard to see how the procedures we have discussed, which often amount to little more than attempts to systematize and further develop the 'measurement' procedures already implied in existing intensive or qualitative work, should have remained controversial and so little used. For these reasons we find arguments about the relative merits of measurement versus non-measurement approaches, survey versus intensive work, and quantitative versus qualitative research unhelpful. Such slogans tend only to divert attention from what we believe is the more fundamental task of creating ideas about the social world in which we can have a reasonable degree of confidence. As we have been arguing, such faith is encouraged by the active consideration of alternative interpretations of research inferences and is reduced by the unthinking use of any technique or a failure formally to concern oneself with the systematic collecting, recording, analyzing, and presenting of data.

We have laboured these strictures about properly conducted social research in relation to the testing of ideas and have continued to maintain a rigid analytic distinction between testing ideas and their initial generation. But, while we would not want to go back on our view that the generation of ideas is possible as the result of any activity or frame of mind, we feel that this distinction, while helping to clarify important issues, is quite unhelpful to the medical sociological enterprise and its division of labour in the practice of research. The generation and testing of ideas are but two *aspects* of work; it is a poor study indeed that does no more than test ideas, just as it is if it merely introduces them.

Glaser and Strauss (1968) have developed the notion of 'theoretical capitalism' to describe the situation where research activity is divided into the generation of ideas (by theoretical capitalists or generals) and those who test them (empirical workers or foot soldiers). We support their reservations about such a division of labour and emphasize the relevance of 'grounded theory' as put forward both by them and by Brown (1973). Grounded theory describes the process whereby ideas and theories are supposedly generated in the ongoing work of systematically testing them. This process is relevant to the refinement of existing theoretical ideas which may go on in each stage of research: design, measurement, and analysis. The process of developing indicators for concepts as described by Brown and Rutter (Reading 1) or of systematically elaborating theories by the consideration of alternative inferences as described by Rosenberg (Reading 4) can itself lead to quite new insights, by focussing attention on the minutiae of phenomenon and on the ambiguities in our theories and ideas as we try to apply them. We feel that more emphasis on the formal testing of ideas against alternatives using the methods outlined above will lead not only to greater confidence in theories in medical sociology but also to the development of new ones.

We have devoted this introduction to a consideration of methodological issues and, by implication, to a criticism of much current work. But we hope that readers of the book will be able to realize that although medical sociology is still at a relatively early stage of development it is a worthwhile and exciting endeavour which has already contributed a great deal both to the practice of medicine and the understanding of the society in which we live.

A note on the editing

The readings are arranged in sections which broadly correspond to the chapter headings in *An Introduction to Medical Sociology*. We have omitted as a special section the Organization of health care but have included two contributions relevant to this topic under the last heading: Medicine and society. The section headings are convenient if somewhat arbitrary. One unfortunate result, however, is that some frequently discussed issues are somewhat hidden. Thus, the topic of professionalization has no formal heading to itself. Readers will note nonetheless that contributions in many parts of the volume are relevant.

Without editing, this book would be two to three times as long. We have, therefore, had to cut many of the papers and we would now like to give some indication of our strategy.

In general, we have selected certain main points in each article and concentrated on those aspects of the text which bear on them. We have not tried to include every issue dealt with in the original articles or chapters of books. The first thing we did, therefore, was to delete sections of those papers which dealt with several issues and to concentrate on only one or two issues in each paper. We then usually cut out any extensive review of theoretical studies. For example, in Coser's paper (Reading 24) we have removed an interesting discussion of Merton's ideas on anomie and alienation. In Cartwright and O'Brien's paper (Reading 10) we have eliminated an early discussion of the weakness of measures of social class and of the Titmuss–Rein–Alderson debate on social class and the health service. In the extracts from Stimson and Webb's book (Reading 16) we have left out the methodological introduction and the conclusions in order to concentrate on sufficient of their findings to give an idea of their approach. In Brown and Rutter's paper (Reading 1) we have cut most of the paragraphs reviewing various approaches to data-collection and interviewing. In general, we have also cut discussions of other literature to a minimum. We do not feel that any of these alterations improve the articles but we feel that enough of the basic ideas and data remain for the reader to appreciate them.

Some readers will always want to look up the original papers and we hope these extracts will encourage people to do so.

As we have argued, it is necessary in establishing research findings to make many checks to rule out alternative interpretations of them. While we have tried to leave in as much of this activity as will allow the reader to see how authors set about such a task this is also another area where we have had to make cuts. Querido's paper (Reading 19), for instance, included an extensive discussion of alternative interpretations and a complex statistical analysis of the types of distress and types of medical and surgical conditions that might interact. We simply report that this produced negative results. Similarly Brown, Birley, and Wing (Reading 8), carried out many statistical checks and extensively considered the measurement of types of schizophrenic symptomatology. This we deleted. Many of the papers included numerous examples to enable a fuller understanding of the phenomena being described. Where we leave in only one example, as in Zola's paper 'From Person to Patient' (Reading 14) or in Stelling and Bucher's 'Vocabularies of Realism' (Reading 18) there were generally several others. Where we had a choice of examples and some had already been quoted in *An Introduction to Medical Sociology* we have always selected alternatives.

Furthermore, we have usually deleted general methodological introductions describing research settings or details of sampling and statistical techniques. We feel these are rather more well established than other aspects of medical sociological methodology. However, what we have tried to include are indications of the degree of variance explained—for example, how many nurses were alienated—and descriptions of methods of measurement and inference.

We have totally eliminated all acknowledgements that authors made to those that helped them and almost every footnote. This is not because we disagree with the practice but for practical considerations.

Finally we should note that every article appears in its present form with the author's permission (or in the case of Balint and Suchman with the permission of the trustee of their estate). In one or two places the authors and ourselves have approved additions to the text for the purpose of clarifying the shortened version. To keep things tidy we have not normally indicated where we made our cuts or additions.

Above all, we should like to thank all the contributors to this volume. They have been generous in their time and the attitude they have taken to the project. They have been very sensitive and understanding to our needs and constraints in editing their work. No one we approached refused to take part. Of course, the contributors bear no responsibility for the general strategy of the reader.

We should also like to thank David Armstrong, Mary-Geo Boulton, George Brown, Ray Fitzpatrick, Steven Green, Mary Griffin, Margot Jefferys, M'Lou Kevlin, and Alwyn Smith for their comments at different stages of the preparation of the volume. Sherry Zeffert has once more been invaluable throughout.

David Tuckett
Joseph M Kaufert
August, 1977

PART ONE
Sociology as a science

The measurement of family activities and relationships: a methodological study

George W. Brown & Michael L. Rutter*

[*The original of this paper is a very full and densely argued one. For reasons of space this version has been edited in accordance with the editors' general strategy. In particular, the thorough review of the background literature and the detailed and erudite discussion of each research decision have been drastically shortened. Details of the sample are reduced and details of an investigation of the effect of the presence or absence of the respondent's spouse, and of the accuracy of a respondent's assessment of another person's feelings, have been altogether eliminated. The authors are Professor of Sociology and of Child Psychiatry respectively in the UK.*]

For the last three years we have been concerned with the development and testing of research techniques aimed to improve the family interview as a research tool, in which an equal amount of attention has been given to obtaining descriptions of family life and to making direct observations of behaviour shown in the interview itself.

The initial development of the instrument was based on interviews with eighty married couples with children, where one patient had recently contacted a psychiatric service. Two kinds of interview were developed. In one, husband and wife were seen separately, and in the other, they were seen together. In the second stage of the work, a further thirty families were seen in order to check certain aspects of the reliability and validity of the measures. Interviews with the patient alone, the spouse alone, and both together, were carried out with each family, using two different investigators at each interview. The interviews carried out with each partner alone take on average about three to four

* extracted from *Human Relations* (1966) 19: 241–63

hours, usually in two sessions. The first hour is taken up with various aspects of the patient's complaint and the rest with questions about the family's day-to-day life together. The interview with the couple together is shorter. It takes about one hour, is entirely concerned with the family's recent contacts with medical and social services, and is designed to get the couple talking together about neutral topics.

'Objective' interview material involves behaviour and events which for the most part can be readily observed by both husband and wife. In the present study, for example, the measures included: kinship contacts; participation in household tasks; participation in child-care activities; contact of parent with child; leisure activities; sexual intercourse; quarrelling; irritability; conversation between the couple; discussion about specific decisions; disagreements over care of the children; behaviour expected of the children (based on reports of behaviour); and behaviour prohibited to the children (based on reports of behaviour). Most are measurements of frequency. In each case it is possible to obtain accounts from husband and wife, and to use these as a preliminary check of validity.

We have been equally interested in the feelings of family members about each other; for example, their criticism of each other or dissatisfaction with aspects of family life. In research interviews, such 'subjective' material is usually obtained by the use of standard questioning. In interviews of any length, however, such material often arises spontaneously, and much of it consists of actual expression, in contrast to self-reports, of feeling. We have used both kinds of 'subjective' material in the present work: that is

   (i) self-reports of feelings ('I get terribly on edge when he's around');

  (ii) actual expressions of positive or negative feeling, considering the words used, tone of voice, gesture, facial expression, and the like.

It is, of course, possible for both to occur together in the same statement; and either may be made spontaneously or in response to a direct question.

The most obvious reason for error in measuring 'objective' material is that the interviewer fails to communicate what he wants to know, or the respondent is insufficiently motivated to recall material accurately.

Often the investigator does not seem to have made up his mind whether he wants an accurate report of events or an expression of attitude. Questions like 'What do you commonly do when your child disobeys you?' probably reflect attitudes as much as what goes on within the home. Most studies have depended on such general questions, only one or two being devoted to the most complex matters.

There have been, however, a number of exceptions which have involved a move to a more flexible mode of questioning. Richardson, Dohrenwend, and Klein (1965) have argued for the use, in certain circumstances, of what they term the 'non-schedule standardized interview'. In contrast to most research interviews, the wording and ordering of questions are not rigidly laid down in advance. The idea is rejected that standardization can automatically be achieved by the use of identically worded questions in the same sequence. Some questions may be given, but the interviewer relies much more on a list of information required. It is his job to inquire into each area of behaviour until he is satisfied he has obtained the material. In a certain sense, the schedule may be said to be a questionnaire addressed to the interviewer and not to the informant.

We have relied on a somewhat similar approach for collecting 'objective' material. In general, it is assumed that for each measure there is a true answer and the job of the interviewer is to approach this as closely as possible by detailed questioning. General questions are not used and general comments about activities by the informant are treated with considerable caution. It is not uncommon for an account obtained by detailed questioning – about washing-up, shopping, and so on – to give quite a different picture from that made in broad, spontaneous generalizations. We would emphasize two advantages: the concentration of detail helps, by the touching-off of associations, the recall of the total picture; and, as Hoffman (1960) has pointed out, it can also result in the fragmentation of the event described, weakening its Gestalt properties. This can divest the event of much of the emotional meaning it might otherwise have, and sometimes avoid arousing anxiety and like emotions which interfere with recall.

We will now mention briefly a number of specific decisions concerning the measurement of 'objective' material that have arisen in the present work.

First, there is the choice of the time to be covered. The interviewer asks about the last week in detail, and then asks how typical the behaviour in this week was of the three months. For habitual events little extra questioning is necessary. For less regular events, such as taking the child to the doctor, a different approach is used: we ask when the event last occurred. When asking about periods such as the last three months we do not necessarily ask about particular dates. Where possible, the interviewer is encouraged to use events that have meaning for the respondent. If an event such as a holiday, a wedding, or an admission to hospital is found to fall near the three-month mark, questions would be asked in terms of this in order to try to reduce any confusion about dates.

Second, we found that, in order to lessen error, much attention had to be given to definitions and rules of procedure, who were kin, how many meetings constitute a contact, etc.

Third, the interviewer must constantly bear in mind that words such as 'quarrel' can be used in different ways. We try to deal with this by using the informant's words, but at the same time obtaining descriptions of events. These enable the interviewer to judge how the words are being used and whether the events are relevant. 'Quarrelling' may be understood to mean different things but, for our purposes, one of certain kinds of behaviour must be present (such as shouting) for a quarrel to be recorded as such.

A fourth problem concerns the complexity of some of the events. This is largely met by flexibility of questioning. The number of questions that may be asked is unrestricted, and the interviewer is expected to continue until he has obtained a full, self-consistent account of a particular event, or until it is clear that further questioning is unlikely to add more. The judgement of the interviewer is of critical importance here. The interviewer has to try to reconstruct the event by specific and, if necessary, frequent probes. This emphasis on flexibility should not, however, be interpreted as a licence to say anything. There are numerous restrictions, particularly concerning 'leading questions'.

A fifth problem has been given much consideration: that of the co-operation of the informant. We do our best to reduce the likelihood of annoyance in a number of ways. For example, the interviewer has to be constantly on the alert for discrepancies, and it is often necessary to go back over material – no rating can be finally made until the interview is completed. Great care is exercised so as to bring up discrepancies tactfully. Again, the informant will often anticipate matters which, according to the order of the interview schedule, would be asked about at a later point. If he seems keen to talk about these, the interviewer should allow him to do so out of turn, rather than attempt to transfer his attention to something else. For a talkative informant it is often possible to collect the bulk of the information needed for lengthy sections of the schedule with little obvious questioning or guidance.

The measurement of feeling and emotion expressed in the interview

Our approach to the measurement of feeling has been dominated by one observation. In the course of a lengthy interview, respondents quite commonly spontaneously express negative feeling which they have denied in response to a direct question; or fail to express positive feeling which may have been expected from their answers to direct questions. The reasons for such behaviour are obscure. We have the impression that it cannot be seen simply as a matter of holding back socially unacceptable sentiments. The reason may also in part relate to the etiquette surrounding questions of the 'How do you feel?' variety. In everyday life there is a strong tendency to give stereotyped replies in response to greetings such as 'How are you today?'

Whatever the reasons for the phenomena, a principal aim of the present work has been to move away from reliance on self-reports about feelings and to record positive and negative feeling expressed in the interview itself. We decided that ratings should be based on verbal and vocal aspects of speech and have developed rules to take account of both. These lay down that there is only a very limited set of conditions in which 'feeling' may be defined by the verbal content of the speech alone – when, for example, a person clearly states that he dislikes or resents something. Otherwise, vocal aspects of speech must be used as well. The interviewer may also take into account facial expression and gesture, but it is our impression that these factors rarely play a crucial role. In measurement we rely entirely on the judgement of the interviewers. Everyone learns to recognize, more or less accurately, kinds of emotional expression – warmth, criticism, dissatisfaction, and so on. Our intention has been to utilize this basic human skill and, through training, to standardize such intuitive judgements.

We record the expression of both negative and positive feeling. Two types of scale are used. One is simply a count of the number of negative and positive statements and the second is an over-all judgement based on the total interview. A basic rating concerns *critical comments* about the spouse and individual children; there is a count of individual comments as well as an over-all rating of severity. The rating is largely based on consideration of tone of voice. A closely allied measure is that of *dissatisfaction*: eight ratings are made about various aspects of the marriage. Five concern the amount and type of involvement of the spouse in child care, relations with the children, household tasks, communication, and the amount of affection and interest. The other three concern any aspect (with a few exceptions) of leisure, sexual relations, finance, and employment. There is also an over-all score based on the sum of the individual scales. *Hostility* to spouse is rated as present or absent by whether there is evidence of a general attitude of rejection – when the person is criticized for what he is rather than for what he does. *Warmth* is the main measure of positive feeling to spouse and the individual children. Most emphasis is placed on tone of voice and, in particular, on how much sympathy is shown when describing symptoms, handicaps, or the relationship. Lack of concern in describing such matters would tend to reduce the rating. A final rating concerns *positive* remarks about the spouse, that is, favourable comments about personality or performance.

No attempt will be made to describe the scales and their accompanying rules in detail; instead, attention will be given to certain problems that have arisen.

Ways of eliciting expression of feeling have been a major concern. Our approach is radically different from that so far described.

There are two ways of obtaining 'subjective' material. A certain amount of reliance is placed on the use of direct questions about feelings: these must be asked in a standard way and with a limited number of additional probes. Standard questions are asked, for instance, about dissatisfaction with eight aspects of the marriage. In these cases, if the interviewer suspects unexpressed feeling, he is not able to go beyond the standard questions in trying to elicit it. Second, we have already pointed out our reliance on spontaneous comments. There are two sources. In quite lengthy sections of the interview the informant is encouraged to talk about his children and marriage. General questions, such as 'How does he get on with your husband?', have been designed only with this purpose in mind. The interviewer introduces additional neutral probes to complete or amplify descriptions or anecdotes about family life: feelings are often expressed when the informant is talking in general about some-one or an everyday incident in the home. This leads to the other equally important source of spontaneous comment. Since much of the interview is taken up with the relating of day-to-day activities and events, there is plenty of opportunity for a person to make such comments.

We have set up simple rules about what the interviewer should do to encourage spontaneous expression of feelings. We consider it important, early in the interview, to establish that we are interested in feelings as well as in the description of events. This is simply done by showing interest (perhaps only with a 'hmm' or a nod of the head) when negative *or* positive feelings are expressed. It is also sometimes useful at an early stage for the interviewer to question further about remarks that he is not sure about. Only neutral probes such as 'How do you feel about this?' are used, which enable the interviewer to rate the original remark. This kind of additional questioning is largely restricted to the early part of the interview and is of course unnecessary if the interviewer has no doubts about rating the informant's expression of feeling.

A second problem we have already touched on. Inconsistency in the expression of feeling is common, and the rating scales have been designed with this in mind. Because positive and negative feelings are often expressed about the same person, we have not incorporated these dimensions in the same scale. Warmth, for example, is rated quite independently of any criticism or dissatisfaction that may be expressed. All scales run from the absence of a single trait to its presence in marked form.

It is, however, one thing to make rules covering such matters, but another to get the rater to follow them. We have been much concerned with possible distortion through 'halo' effects. In combating this persistent tendency, we rely on two procedures. The use of unipolar scales, we have already mentioned. The other is extensive training. This has a number of features. First, there is a series of detailed definitions and notes. Second, there are 'master' tape-recordings of interviews with accompanying notes, pointing out, for instance, individual critical comments, or illustrating the five levels of over-all severity of criticism towards the spouse. The tapes are particularly important for arriving at common standards for rating of expressed feeling. Third, a new interviewer accompanies more experienced workers on a number of interviews, rates separately, and then discusses discrepancies. Last, weekly meetings are held to discuss problems arising from the work.

Thirty families were seen. The study was designed to make two basic kinds of comparison. First, a comparison of the ratings made by the two investigators present at the same interview. This constitutes a *within*-interview comparison to test whether investigators can agree on ratings based on the same material. The second comparison is *across*-interview – that is, between agreed ratings based on different material, between the spouse interview and the patient interview, or between either of these and the joint interview. Such comparisons largely concern the validity of the material.

All families were told that the work was for research purposes, that all information would be treated confidentially, and that nothing would be passed on to the other spouse.

Suitable families living in South London were approached as they came into contact with psychiatric services.

Three questions will be considered:

Table 1 *Agreement between raters present at the same interview: feelings expressed about marital partner*

	no. of scale points	single interview agreement (N = 60)	joint interview agreement (N = 36)
warmth	6	0.79	0.85
number of positive remarks	—	0.85	*
severity of criticism	5	0.90	0.89
number of critical remarks	—	0.89	0.84
dissatisfaction (eight scales)	4	range 0.78–0.95 mean 0.84	*
total score of dissatisfaction	25	0.95	*
hostility	2	98%	97%

* not rated in joint interview

Table 2 *Agreement between raters present at the same interview Summary scales of relationships (selected scales)*

	Pearson r (N = 60)	no. of scale points
marital relationship	0.82	4
tension in the home	0.86	4
strain of patient and strain of spouse with parents (own report)	0.93	3
strain of patient and strain of spouse with parents (as reported by other person)	0.87	3

1 Can trained investigators agree in their judgements about feelings expressed by the informant towards his spouse or children?
Table 1 shows that the amount of agreement between investigators present at the same interview about the rating of expressed feelings is high, and that the results for the single and joint interviews are similar – the average product moment correlation is 0.85. Similar results are obtained when spouse and patient ratings are analyzed separately.

2 Can reliable over-all judgements be made about the quality of relationships?
Table 2 shows that raters show much the same levels of agreement for the summary scales of relationships, which take account of all information in the interview. Correlations range from 0.81 to 0.91.

3 Do husbands and wives when seen separately give comparable accounts of family activities?

This third question concerns the *across*-interview comparison of the 'objective' material. First, a mention should be made of the interrater reliability of these 'objective measures'. Most of the correlations between raters are between 0.90 and 0.95. The only ones that fall a little below this are those concerned with irritability, where somewhat more judgement is involved. Those concerning the informant's account of irritability towards his or her spouse and child are 0.80 and 0.87 respectively, and those concerned with the informant's account of his spouse's irritability to the informant and child are 0.82 and 0.90 respectively. These results are not surprising. Considerable attention had been given to the definitions of the various results. It should be added, however, that some studies have reported considerably lower interrater agreement for activity measures.

The *across*-interview level of agreement between the separate accounts of husband and wife in the single interviews posed further questions. *Table 3* (see over) gives a representative selection of results. It shows that, for the three months before interview, the majority of correlations are over 0.60 and many are between 0.70 and 0.80. Measures concerned with kinship contacts, participation of husband and wife in child care and household tasks, positive interaction with the selected child, behaviour expected of and prohibited to the child, disagreement over child rearing, and leisure activities all reach satisfactory levels of agreement.

Irritability, quarrelling, and the like proved difficult areas of behaviour to measure, and in the first twenty interviews the level of the *across*-interview agreement was only modest. Group discussion about interviewing technique, accompanied by a tightening of definitions, led to a very marked improvement in the agreement between the separate accounts of husband and wife. The final correlations for the thirty cases are almost all in the 0.60 to 0.70 range. That for quarrelling, however, reached only 0.43, but we have some reason to believe that in future work this can be improved.

In common with a few other workers who have looked at the matter, we find that the measurement of communication and decision-making by such interviewing is unsatisfactory.

Two major reasons for agreement being only moderately good on certain measures suggest themselves. The first concerns the relation between feelings about the activity and the accuracy with which they are reported. Sherif and Hovland (1961) note that effects on the reporting of information have not yet been studied experimentally, but consider that consistent biases would occur – that where topics were associated

Table 3   *Across-interview agreement between marital partners about activities (selected scales)*

	3-month period before interview (N = 30)	3-month period 1 year before interview (N = 20)[b]
total range kin contacts of patient	0.91	not asked
frequency of kin contacts of patient with own kin	0.92	not asked
participation in household tasks of wife	0.67	0.60
participation in household tasks of husband	0.75	0.54
positive interaction of spouse with child[a]	0.78	0.79
positive interaction of patient with child[a]	0.72	0.66
disagreement of parents over child-rearing[a]	0.68	not asked
behaviour expected of child by parent[a]	0.69	not asked
behaviour prohibited to child by parents[a]	0.62	not asked
communication of spouse with child[a]	0.67	not asked
communication of patient with child[a]	0.45	not asked
leisure activity of patient and spouse together	0.72	0.54
leisure activity of spouse alone	0.60	0.60
leisure activity of patient alone	0.42	0.28
amount of nagging between husband and wife	0.61	0.16
irritability of patient to spouse	0.67	0.26
irritability of patient to child	0.58	0.17
amount of quarrelling in home	0.43	0.11
frequency of sexual intercourse	0.36	0.53
amount of discussion about decisions	0.48[b]	not asked
everyday conversation between couple	0.16[b]	not asked

[a] Families with no children over 3 were excluded from these measures.
[b] N = 20. These measures were not made on the final ten families.

with strong feeling there would be a shift in reporting in a systematic direction. As far as the reporting of family activities in the present study is concerned, such a 'displacement effect' would seem most likely to be measurable where both husband and wife have full knowledge of the activity and where expressed feelings tend to relate to the frequency rather than to some qualitative aspect of performance of the spouse. These conditions hold for reporting by the wife about her husband's participation in child care and household tasks (seventeen items of behaviour were covered in detail). In the areas of both household tasks and child care, dissatisfied wives tend to report less participation than their husbands, and the wives who did not express dissatisfaction much the same or a little more. *Table 4* shows this material in its simplest form, by whether the wife reports more of less than her husband.

Table 4   *Comparison of husband's and wife's accounts of husband's participation in household tasks and child care, by whether wife is dissatisfied with husband's participation in these areas*

		wife reports more than husband	wife reports less than husband	p
household tasks	wife dissatisfied	4	8	p < 0.05
	wife not dissatisfied	13	3	
child care	wife dissatisfied	1	4	p > 0.10
	wife not dissatisfied	6	8	
total	wife dissatisfied	5	12	p > 0.05
	wife not dissatisfied	19	11	

notes: (i) scale 0 to 100: 100 = everything done by husband
(ii) families with no children under 11 were excluded from 'child care'
(iii) 3 cases of complete agreement excluded

Conclusion

Thus we have shown that an interview and rating scale measuring a wide range of aspects of family life can be developed and can lead to the reliable collection of data regarding feelings and activities in the home.

If investigators are trained to recognize and rate the expression of emotions using carefully established procedures and definitions, high levels of agreement can be achieved among them. Such procedures require a special approach involving detailed questioning of respondents which is quite different to the schedule interviewing approach common in so many studies.

Our study of *across*-interviewee agreement shows first that it is possible to confirm accounts of activities in the home by speaking to both people involved. However, in certain areas of family life emotions can play a strong part in influencing the reporting of activities. Thus, satisfied and dissatisfied wives, respectively, appeared to exaggerate or underplay their husband's role in housework or child care. Such factors make a flexible interviewing technique essential. It is most unlikely that we could have obtained accurate and reliable accounts using the more traditional schedule interview technique. Such an instrument will tend to pick up attitudes and emotions rather than accurate accounts of behaviour.

We suggest that the kind of flexible interviewing technique we have described, assigning a large role to the interviewer's skill, judgement, and human capacities, can provide valid data in areas of complexity or strong feelings and that, given adequate training and time to develop clear procedures, it will not do so at the risk of low reliability.

2   The measurement of expressed emotion in the families of psychiatric patients

Christine Vaughn & Julian Leff*

[*This paper has been reduced from the original by only a small amount in accordance with the editors' general strategy. The authors are a psychologist in the USA and a consultant psychiatrist in the UK, respectively.*]

In a series of studies of the influence of family life on the course of an established schizophrenic illness, it has been shown that the level of emotion expressed by relatives shortly after a schizophrenic patient is admitted to hospital is strongly associated with symptomatic relapse during the nine months following discharge (Brown, Birley, and Wing 1972; see Reading 8). This paper describes a modification of the primary research instrument used in these studies, the Camberwell family interview schedule, described by Brown and Rutter (Brown and Rutter 1966; see Reading 1), which shortens the interview to less than half of its original length without affecting the predictive value of the expressed emotion scales. Although shown to be a reliable and valid instrument, the original family interview sometimes took as long as four or five hours to administer. This could be a taxing exercise for both interviewer and informant, and usually two separate visits were required in order to complete the schedule. Every conceivable aspect of family life was

* extracted from the *British Journal of Social and Clinical Psychology* (1976a) **15**: 157–65.

covered. Since the factors most closely associated with symptomatic relapse of schizophrenia were not known at the time of the 1972 study, it seemed desirable then to elicit as much information as possible about potentially relevant areas. Also, it seemed likely that it might be necessary to question someone for quite a while, perhaps several hours, before rapport was such that the person would be willing to give an honest account of his feelings. This was a most important point, since a primary purpose of the schedule, as designed by Brown and Rutter (see Reading 1), was to provide material from which ratings of emotional response could be made. But if these same ratings could be made on the basis of a shorter interview, this would of course be preferable. Some people would be spared an exhausting ordeal and later investigators interested in the technique for research purposes would not be deterred by its sheer length.

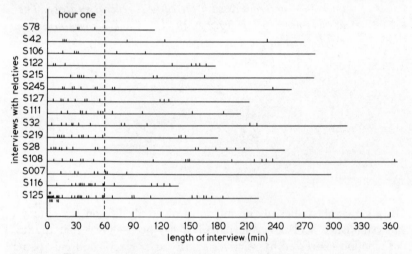

Figure 1   The occurrence of critical comments during 15 interviews with key relatives of schizophrenic patients in the Brown, Birley, and Wing (1972) study. Each horizontal line represents the length of an interview with a key relative of a patient, identified by the project case number to the left of the line. The short vertical lines represent individual units of criticism or 'critical' comments as defined by Brown, Birley, and Wing (1972).

As the number of critical comments made by the relative about the patient was the crucial measure in predicting symptomatic relapse, it seemed desirable to listen to tape-recorded interviews from the original study in order to determine the point in time when, and the area of inquiry in which, critical comments occurred. If the main criticism occurred in the early stages of the interview or during some other specific stage, a judiciously abbreviated interview might well be justified.

In cases where all critical remarks had been recorded by the interviewer on the rating summary, it was necessary only to listen to each tape and to note at which points individual criticisms occurred and which topics were being covered at the time. Fifteen interviews were listened to in this way, with equal representation of high, medium, and low criticism interviews. Individual time graphs were then plotted (*Figure 1*).

The results were remarkably consistent. The three sections of the interview which deal with psychiatric history, irritability and quarrelling, and clinical symptoms in the three-month pre-admission period accounted for 67 per cent of all critical remarks over fifteen interviews. It is difficult to know whether topic or primacy of questioning was responsible for this finding, since these same three sections were also the first three areas covered in almost every interview. Furthermore, in the first part of the interview the interviewer would sometimes allow the relative to talk freely about the patient until it seemed possible to begin questioning in a more systematic way. He might follow up individual areas of questioning earlier than usual if brought up spontaneously by the relative. In any event, the majority of critical comments were produced within the first hour, and there was virtually no relationship between total number of critical comments and length of interview ($r = 0.08$). Criticism occurred particularly during detailed questioning about the development of the illness and the patient's present clinical condition. What was surprising was that once certain areas were covered, later sections (with the exception of household tasks/money matters and, in the case of parental households only, relationships) produced very little criticism relative to the total amount. Kinship, for example – a lengthy section about which questioning often continued for as long as an hour – accounted for only 0.5 per cent of all critical remarks over the fifteen interviews. The marital relationship section, which probes such potentially critical areas as leisure activities and the amount of affection and interest between patient and spouse, contributed only 3 per cent of all critical comments. This is not to say that patients were never criticized for their performance as husbands or wives; they frequently were. The point is that if such criticism occurred at all, it was brought out spontaneously early on in the interview, and not during the direct questioning about the marital relationship.

These results supported the use of a shortened interview in which the areas most likely to produce any criticism were given priority in the sequence of questioning. In practice, only minimal reordering was required. The household tasks/money matters and relationship sections now follow the psychiatric history, irritability/quarrelling, and clinical

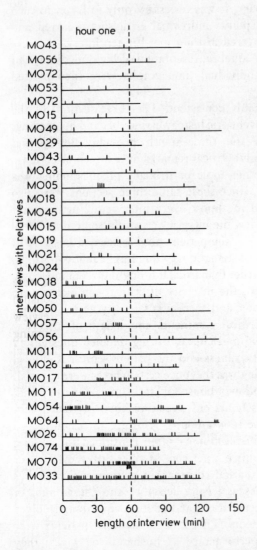

Figure 2 The occurrence of critical comments during 32 interviews with the key relatives of 25 schizophrenic patients in the present study. In cases where a patient's parents were seen and both were critical, a project number appears twice. An additional interview with a critical relative (MO22) was excluded from this analysis, as the interview was not tape-recorded. Interviews in which there was no criticism are not shown ($n = 13$).

symptoms sections. A few additional sections have been retained in order to make other required ratings such as amount of face-to-face contact and drug-taking. Once these sections are covered, however, questioning ceases. The present abbreviated version takes from one to two hours to administer. The form and content of the questions in each section and the relevant rating scales are unchanged.

Findings in the present study provide striking support for the usefulness of the abbreviated interview in predicting symptomatic relapse in schizophrenic patients in the nine months following discharge from hospital. It has proved possible not only to replicate the results of Brown, Birley, and Wing (1972) with a different group of schizophrenic patients, but also to predict relapse patterns even more precisely than in the earlier study. These results are reported elsewhere (Vaughn and Leff 1976b).

A consideration of the occurrence of criticism during interviews with forty-six relatives of schizophrenic patients reveals response patterns which are very similar to those shown by the sample of fifteen from the 1972 study (*Figure 2*). In the thirty-three interviews in which a relative was at all critical the number of critical remarks made bore only a negligible relationship to the interview's length ($r = 0.24$), which in the present study varied from one to two hours with a mean length of one hour forty-five minutes. Critical remarks, if any, tended to occur during the first hour of the interview.

Another way of showing that the amount of criticism produced is unrelated to the length of interview is to compare the mean number of critical remarks made by the relatives of the two series of schizophrenic patients. The mean number of comments made by the forty-six relatives in the present study was 8.22 (S.D. = 11.11). The mean number of comments for all 126 relatives interviewed in the 1972 study was 7.86 (S.D. = 14.40). Statistically, these two findings are not significantly different ($z = 0.173$), despite the great differences in length of interview in the two studies.

Our original intention had been to cut down the length of the rather cumbersome family interview to no more than two hours without impairing its predictive validity. Having achieved this aim successfully we were then led to ask whether a further reduction in its length to no more than one hour was possible. This possibility was examined by comparing the rank ordering of the interviews based on the number of critical comments produced in the first hour with that based on the total number of remarks produced during the entire interview. The correlation coefficient between these two rank orderings was found to be 0.90. This result indicates that if the sole purpose of the interview were to rank the relatives on the basis of criticism voiced, it would be unnecessary to prolong it beyond one hour.

The high correlation found in this group of relatives of schizophrenic patients, between the number of criticisms in the first hour and the number in the whole interview, could result from several different distributions of critical comments. We have already seen from *Figures 1* and *2* that the critical comments of relatives of schizophrenic patients, both in the study of Brown, Birley, and Wing (1972) and in our own, show a distribution skewed towards the beginning of the interview. This pattern is reflected in the low correlations between number of critical comments and length of interview (0.08 in the study of Brown, Birley,

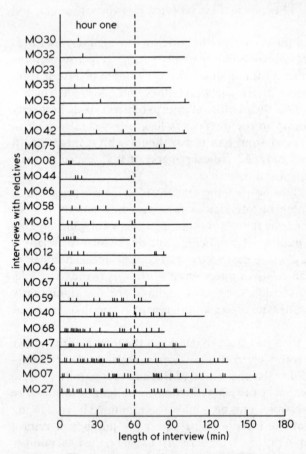

Figure 3   The occurrence of critical comments during 24 interviews with the key relatives of 24 depressed neurotic patients in the present study. Interviews in which there was no criticism are not shown (*n* = 8).

and Wing and 0.24 in our study). But the group of relatives of neurotic depressive patients in our study provides a marked contrast with the relatives of schizophrenic patients. The mean number of total critical remarks made does not differ significantly for the two groups of relatives (mean $= 7.19$, S.D. $= 9.86$, depressed group; mean $= 8.22$, S.D. $= 11.11$, schizophrenic group; $t = 0.422$, 76 d.f.). The relatives of the depressed patients also show a high correlation (0.95) between the rank ordering based on the number of critical comments in the first hour and that based on the total number of such remarks. However, there is no dropping off in criticism after the first hour, as in the schizophrenic group. As shown in *Figure 3*, there is a steady rate of expression of critical comments, which is reflected in a highly significant correlation between number of criticisms and length of interview (0.64, $p < 0.001$). This interesting and unexpected difference between relatives of schizophrenic and depressed neurotic patients will be explored further in a subsequent paper. At present, it is sufficient to state that in the case of both groups of relatives it is possible to achieve a representative measure of their critical attitudes on the basis of the first hour of the interview alone.

3   An appraisal with implications
for theoretical development
of some epidemiological work
on heart disease

*Edward A. Suchman**

[*This paper is complete. The author was an early and
distinguished pioneer of medical sociology in the USA.*]

Marks's (1967) paper [reviewing epidemiological research on heart
disease] substantiates a well-known fact in social research: nothing is
as sterile as demographic group comparisons. Rates analyzed in relation
to such categories as sex, age, race, marital status, occupation, and
geographical region are an essential part of the social book-keeping of
modern society. In and of themselves, however, these rates offer little
by way of explanation. If one's purpose is to explain the relation
between demographic factors and coronary heart disease, one cannot
help but get lost in a morass of inconclusive correlations. Even if the
definitions and methods were good – as they often are not – the results
would still be inconclusive. The task of seeking to verify causal
hypotheses such as the present one on chronic emotional stress and

* extracted from the *Millbank Memorial Fund Quarterly* (1967) **XIV** (2) part 2:
109–13, April. This paper was originally delivered as a contribution to a symposium
on social stress and cardiovascular disease held in Phoenix, Arizona, USA, February
14–16, 1966.

coronary heart disease via the route of demographic group comparisons is a difficult one. It can only bog down, as Marks's painstaking analysis has shown so well, in a minimum of understanding and a maximum of methodological dispute.

The task of this paper is to appraise Marks's (1967) review of empirical findings in an attempt to further theoretical development. Marks has struggled valiantly with hundreds of disconnected statistical correlations between demographic characteristics and the prevalence and incidence of coronary heart disease. Never have so many said so little.

Both theoretically and methodologically the primary task appears on the surface to be simple enough. Look at existing morbidity and mortality statistics for coronary heart disease and compare the rates for different demographic groups. For the purposes of this conference, Marks has not even challenged, which she could easily have done, existing measures of either coronary heart disease or the major demographic variables. In her review of research findings, only rarely was she able to insert chronic emotional stress as one of the crucial variables under consideration. Yet, despite the simplicity of the research problem, the over-all impression gained from her review is one of an overwhelming epidemiological infarct.

Where does the fault lie? The answer is probably to be found in the essential meaningfulness of gross, demographic population categories when viewed as 'causal' variables indicative of social processes. These may be convenient, easily studied labels for subdividing populations, but they are not dynamic social ideas and cannot, except in a very limited, superficial sense, represent the kind of social phenomena that may cause disease or anything else.

Marks clearly indicates the great need to move beyond these descriptive population labels to research upon causal hypotheses. Social research made this transition many years ago. One of the best pieces of social epidemiology was done before either epidemiology or sociology achieved its present status or financial support. This was Durkheim's (1952) analysis of suicide rates by social groupings. Durkheim placed the emphasis where it belonged – on the study of the social process underlying the observed differences. He was not primarily concerned with the Japanese or the French as nationalities. Further, he studied suicides not as a category in mortality tables, but as a meaningful and productive vehicle for observing the effects of group integration. Imagine being interested in coronary artery disease today only because it was a good way of studying chronic emotional stress. If this is not so, however, the fault lies largely with the sociologists and psychologists for having neglected disease as a social phenomenon.

In his remarks on Smith's (1967) paper, Cassel (1967) challenged the traditional model of disease causation, especially insofar as social factors were involved. He offered an approach which attempted to avoid circularity of definition and to provide for more direct study of the causal process. These two problems of stating cause and effect relationships of variables which represent independent phenomena and of identifying the intervening steps between cause and effect, as directly as possible, are the backbone of current sociological research methods. This is the direction in which future research on social factors in disease must go if it is to break out of the current stranglehold of traditional epidemiology.

Some of the basic and crucial principles of design and analysis should be summarized briefly since they are often absent in much current epidemiological research. Begin where any piece of research must – with a hypothesis that relates two variables, one independent or 'antecedent-causal', and the other dependent or 'consequent-effect'. This antecedent-consequent relationship, however, is only the starting point of the research process – not its end, despite the impression given by Marks's review. In and of itself, such an hypothesis is largely meaningless. Meaning can come only as one attempts to explain this relationship in terms of other variables in the causal sequence, of which the observed relationship is but one segment.

Research on social factors as 'causes', whether of heart disease, suicide, or voting, begins with the notion of an unlimited series of related events all of which have multiple causes and in turn produce multiple effects. This on-going chain of related events may be conceived as having no 'original' cause or 'ultimate' effect and of being subject to an infinite number of intervening events. Out of this universe of interrelationships the researcher may select any two events as the basis for his working hypothesis. One event (the earlier in time) he will arbitrarily label as his independent or hypothesized causal variable, while the other (the later in time) becomes his dependent or hypothesized effect variable. The selection of which two events to relate, of course, springs largely from existing theory and knowledge as applied to the problem being investigated. Obviously, what serves as the independent variable in one study may become the dependent variable in another study depending upon the segment of the causal chain selected for research.

The first step in the research process following the development of a working hypothesis relating two events in an antecedent-consequent relationship, is the establishment of a significant association between the two. Finding such an association, one is now in a position both to test the validity of this association and to elaborate upon it in terms of other events in the causal sequence either preceding, intervening, or following. This sequence might be diagrammed as follows, keeping in mind the arbitrariness of defining any two variables as independent or dependent. Preceding variables (preconditions) – independent variable (cause) – intervening variables (modifiers) – dependent variable (effect) – following variables (consequences).

Given this model, one may ask such analytical questions as:

1 What is the relationship between the cause and effect variables?
2 To what extent is this relationship attributable to or modified by some precondition variable?
3 How does this relationship come about in terms of intervening variables which permit, modify, or condition the relationship?
4 What are the consequences of this relationship in terms of the events that follow?

Seeking the answers to questions such as these constitutes a large part of what is called the social research process. Many of the questions raised in the discussions of heart disease about contextual analyses, conditional relationships, and internal and external factors could easily fit into this basic model of social research.

In appraisal of the review of findings offered by Marks, very rarely did any of the studies go beyond the statement of the relationship between some demographic factor and coronary heart disease. The discovery of such a relationship does not answer any questions regarding social causation. Until the observed relationship is broken down further by some third variable, it can be neither explained, nor interpreted, nor elaborated.

A wide variety of sociological and psychological variables could be introduced as intervening variables into the reported correlations between such factors as sex, age, education, race, nationality, religion, occupation and income, and coronary heart disease. These intervening variables must, after all, be of the same nature as those used to explain correlations between demographic characteristics and any other social phenomenon. One could certainly conceive of some original schemes for linking these factors to coronary heart disease, but a new mouse trap need not be invented when so many tried-and-true models have not even been touched in this area of research. As has been pointed out, the epidemiological studies of such important social phenomena as status inconsistency have hardly approached the sophistication of research on these variables in relation to phenomena other than disease.

In conclusion, the following exercise is offered. Consider any major study of some sociological dependent variable, such as prejudice, voting behaviour, or adjustment to the Army. Observe the rather minor role which comparisons by sex, age, and occupation have in the analysis. Note the tremendous concern with introducing and interpreting the intervening variables. If the study is a longitudinal one, the ubiquitous fourfold table becomes sixteenfold. The search becomes, clearly one of trying to find out why A relates to B, by way of introducing C and D, and E and F. Where are these test variables in epidemiological research?

4   The use of test factors to assess the relationship between variables

*Morris Rosenberg**

[*This reading is taken from a book dealing with the logical principles underlying data analysis procedures; for purposes of simplicity, sub-group classification is used. This short extract illustrates how one deals with the problem of spuriousness. The author is Professor of Sociology at the University of Maryland, USA.*]

The sociologist is characteristically interested in the relationship of social experience to individual mental processes and acts. He thus tends to select as his independent variable certain groups, collectivities, or social categories and chooses as his dependent variable socially relevant opinions, attitudes, values, or actions. Thus he may ask: Are workers more alienated than middle-class people? Do Catholics vote democratic more than Protestants? Are older people more prejudiced than younger people? Are small town youngsters less likely to go on to college than city dwellers? And so on.

Given proper sample and research design, the analyst may be able to provide correct answers to these questions. But these results are essentially descriptive. They may show that Catholics vote democratic more than Protestants do, but they do not indicate why this is so. While it is valuable to explain such a relationship on the basis of informed

*extracted from Morris Rosenberg, *The Logic of Survey Analysis* (1966) New York: Basic Books: 23–36.

speculation, it is still more valuable to subject this speculation to a systematic test. The most important systematic way of examining the relationship between two variables is to introduce a third variable, called a test factor, into the analysis. This is what is meant by the process of *elaboration*.

The test factor, it should be stressed, is introduced solely for the purpose of increasing one's understanding of the original two-variable relationship. The aim of the analysis is to determine whether the relationship between X (the independent variable) and Y (the dependent variable) is due to Z (the test factor).

But what is meant by saying that the relationship is 'due to' Z, or that Z is 'responsible for' or the 'determinant of' the relationship between X and Y? In the present discussion, these terms have a rather definite meaning. To say that the relationship between X and Y is due to Z is to mean that *were it not for* Z, there would be *no* relationship between X and Y. The statement, 'Catholics have lower suicide rates because they are more integrated', must be translated as, 'Were Catholics not more integrated, they would not have lower suicide rates'. Similarly, 'Lower-class people have higher rates of schizophrenia because they are more socially isolated' is translated as, 'Were lower-class people not more socially isolated, they would not have higher rates of schizophrenia'.

The procedural aspect of the key phrase 'were it not for' is to *control on*, or *hold constant*, the test factor, thereby eliminating its influence on the relationship. Let us consider how one 'holds constant' a test factor by means of the technique of *sub-group classification*.

Assume we begin with the finding that older people are more likely than younger people to listen to religious programs on the radio (*Table 5*). In considering why this may be so, we suggest that perhaps this is due to the factor of education. Translated: were older people not more poorly educated, then they would not be more likely to listen to religious programs.

The task, then, is to eliminate the influence of education. This can be done simply by comparing older and younger people of *equal education*. Thus, one compares the listening habits of *well-educated* and *poorly-educated* old and young people. *Table 6* shows the results.

We see that among the well educated, older people are hardly more likely to listen to religious programmes, and the same is true among poorly-educated people. Thus, were it not for education, there would be almost no relationship between age and listening. These data thus point to the following conclusion: older people are more likely to listen to religious programs because older people are generally more poorly

Table 5   *Age and listening to religious programs*

listen to religious programs	young listeners	old listeners
yes	17%	26%
no	83	74
total per cent	100	100

Source: Lazarsfeld and Rosenberg (1955: 117)

educated and poorly-educated people are more likely to listen to religious programs.

This analytic process may be expressed more generally by means of technical terminology. Typically one begins with a relationship between an independent variable (age) and a dependent variable (religious program listening). One then seeks to explain this relationship by introducing an explanatory variable, called a test factor (education). The method used is to *stratify* on the test factor and to examine the contingent

Table 6   *Age and listening to religious program by education*

listen to religious programs	high education		low education	
	young	old	young	old
yes	9%	11%	29%	32%
no	91	89	71	68
total per cent	100	100	100	100

source: Lazarsfeld and Rosenberg (1955: 117)

associations. 'Stratification' means that we have broken the test factor into its component categories. In this case it is highly educated and poorly educated; in other cases it might be men and women, or Catholics, Protestants, and Jews, or upper, middle, and lower classes, etc.

The process of stratification creates 'contingent associations'. In *Table 6*, two contingent associations appear. The first is the association between age and program listening among the well educated; the second is the association between age and listening among the poorly educated. If the test factor has more categories (say, grammar school education, high school education, college education, and postgraduate education) then there will be more contingent associations – one for each category. If the relationship between age and listening disappears within each contingent association, then we can say that the relationship is due to the test factor (education).

In order to understand the relationship between two variables, then, it is necessary to introduce additional variables into the analysis. But which variables should these be? In order to answer this question, it is necessary to digress momentarily to discuss a peculiar but decisive characteristic of sociological variables, namely, the fact that they are 'block-booked'.

The concept of block-booking is drawn from the field of mass communications research. At an earlier period in the history of the film industry, it was customary for film producers to rent films to exhibitors *en masse*, for example, in blocks of five. Thus an exhibitor had the option of renting or not renting a block of five films, but could not choose among them. If the block contained, say, one highly desirable film, one fairly desirable film, and three undesirable films, the exhibitor was compelled to take the undesirable films in order to obtain the desirable ones.

Human beings (or other sociological units) are similarly 'block-booked'. Each man (or group, or region) may be characterized in terms of a number of dimensions. When we describe a man in terms of certain characteristics, we are at the same time describing him in terms of other characteristics.

Let us say that we find that blue-collar workers are more alienated than white-collar workers. But blue-collar workers differ from white-collar workers in many ways other than in the type of work they do. They tend to be more poorly educated; they are more likely to be Catholic; they are more likely to be liberal on economic issues and illiberal on social issues; they are less likely to engage in abstract modes of thought; they are less likely to have high IQs; they are more likely to come from large families; and so on.

'Blue-collar', then, means a great many things. When we try to explain why blue-collar workers are more alienated, then, we do so by giving consideration to these other factors associated with the status of blue-collar worker. It is these 'block-booked', or associated, characteristics which enable us to understand why blue-collar workers are more alienated. The aim of the analysis is to ascertain *what there is* about being a blue-collar worker which accounts for the relationship with alienation.

Block-booking is the central fact of survey analysis. One cannot properly understand the relationship between an independent and a dependent variable without taking account of the fact that other variables are associated with them. These associated variables become the 'test factors'.

But not all test factors have the same meaning, serve the same theoretical purpose, or have the same statistical properties. At least six types of test factors may be distinguished: extraneous variables, component variables, intervening variables, antecedent variables, suppressor variables, and distorter variables. The purpose of this discussion is to suggest how these types of test factors enable one to achieve sounder, more precise, and more meaningful interpretations of two-variable relationships.

Extraneous variables

When a research investigator discovers a relationship between two variables, the first question he implicitly asks is: 'Is it real?' Knowing that sociological variables are 'block-booked', he is concerned to know whether there is an *inherent link* between the independent and dependent variables or whether it is based on an accidental connection with some associated variable. In short, he must guard against what are called 'spurious relationships'.

Strictly speaking, there is no such thing as a spurious relationship; there are only spurious interpretations. It is customary to use the term 'spurious relationship', however, to refer to a case in which there is no meaningful or inherent link between the two variables; the relationship is due solely to the fact that each of the variables happens accidentally to be associated with some other variable.

The point is obvious when one considers gross examples. A common favorite is the finding that in Sweden there is a relationship between the number of storks in an area and the number of children born in the area. One calls this relationship spurious, even though there is nothing spurious about the relationship; what is spurious is the *interpretation* that the storks bring the babies.

In the above example, the reason for the original relationship is always some associated third variable. The reason for the relationship between number of storks and number of babies is rural-urban location. Most storks are found in rural areas and the rural birth rate is higher than the urban birth rate.

Unless one guards against such accidental associations, one is in danger of reaching erroneous and misleading conclusions. The significance of this point for sociological theory is apparent. Much ingenious and suggestive speculation, leading to important theoretical conclusions, may be advanced to explain certain empirical relationships, when the truth of the matter lies in the fact that an accidental link binds the independent and dependent variables. Without such a check, there may enter into the body of sociological theory ideas which are erroneous but which may exert a wide influence in the field.

No one, of course, will be deceived by the examples cited above. But let us consider some more serious illustrations. In each case we start with a relationship between two variables, we speculate on the meaning of this relationship, and we find that our interpretations are erroneous and misleading by virtue of our failure to take account of extraneous variables.

Example

A striking example of the theoretical importance of considering control variables appears in a study by Goldhamer and Marshall (1949). In their book, *Psychosis and Civilization*, they undertook to examine the widely held assumption that rates of psychosis had increased over the last century. And, in fact, the data did show a striking and consistent rise. It would not be difficult to suggest some of the changing conditions of life which created intensified stress and which might be responsible for mental breakdown: the increased mobility aspirations which were largely frustrated; the shift from the farm to the city, substituting the isolation and anonymity of urban living for the social integration of rural life; the breakdown in the stabilizing force of religion; the heightened competitiveness of economic life; the development of urban slums; the increased anomie of a swiftly changing and socially mobile society; the breakdown of the stability of the family expressed in increased rates of divorce, etc. All these factors represented theoretical bases for accounting for the observed rise in the rate of psychosis.

Goldhamer and Marshall noted that the increased rates of hospitalization for psychosis between 1845 and 1945, however, failed to take account of the factor of *age*. If one examined the rates of psychosis within each age category, one found (with the exception of those over fifty) that *there was virtually no change over the century-long period*. The relationship was largely a spurious one.

How did age produce this misleading interpretation? The most common psychosis of advanced age is senile dementia; this is primarily an organic (rather than a functional) psychosis and is more often due to physiological degeneration than to psychological stress. Now, the advances in medicine during the period 1845–1945 had produced an increase in average length of life of the population. Hence, the proportion of old people in the population was much greater in the later period, thus producing a very large *number* of people with senile dementia. There has also been 'an increased tendency to hospitalize persons suffering from the mental diseases of the senium'. Hence, the higher total rate of psychosis in 1945 was largely a reflection of the changing age distribution of the population and a tendency to hospitalize older people, not a reflection of increased societal stress (except perhaps among older people).

This is a striking illustration of how an elaborate and sophisticated theoretical structure might have been constructed to account for a relationship which was, in fact, completely misleading by virtue of the failure to take account of an extraneous variable.

The method of determining whether one has made a misleading interpretation is to control on the test factor. If, when the influence of the extraneous test factor is held constant, one finds that the relationship disappears, then it may be concluded that the relationship is due to the extraneous variable. If one is to avoid drawing erroneous or misleading conclusions from data, therefore, it is essential to guard against such accidental links.

Support of an interpretation

Just as test factors may be introduced to show that highly plausible interpretations are actually misleading, so may they provide evidence that highly dubious interpretations are actually sound. An investigation of the relationship between parental interest and adolescent self-esteem affords a case in point.

Table 7 *Reports of mother's knowledge of child's friends and subject's self-esteem*

respondent's self-esteem	'During this period (age 10 or 11) did your mother know who most of your friends were?'		
	all or most	some or none	don't know or can't remember
high	46%	32%	27%
medium	23	25	38
low	30	43	35
total per cent	100	100	100
number	(1407)	(133)	(26)

source: Rosenberg (1963: 38)

In this study, adolescents were requested to think back to the period when they were about ten or eleven years old and were asked, 'During this period [age ten or eleven] did your mother know who most of your friends were?' *Table 7* (see back) shows that the more friends known by the mother, according to the respondent's report, the larger the proportion with high self-esteem.

However, one is immediately suspicious of such a finding. It is entirely possible that the child who dislikes, or gets on poorly with, his mother will 'remember' her as showing little interest in, or knowledge of, people who were important to him at an earlier age. In this case, the relationship might simply reflect the fact that adolescents with unfavorable attitudes towards their mothers say that their mothers did not know their friends, and these people also tend to have low self-esteem. The task, then, is to control on unfavorable attitude towards mothers in order to see whether the relationship then vanishes.

One question which partly reflects the student's present attitude towards his mother is, 'When your parents disagree, whose side are you usually on – your mother's or your father's?' *Table 8* shows that whether the adolescent says he is usually on his mother's side or usually on his

Table 8 *Reports of mother's knowledge of child's friends and subject's self-esteem by identification with parents*

	student currently identifies chiefly with ...					
	mother		*father*		*both equally*	
	mother knew friends ...					
respondent's self-esteem	*all or most*	*some or none*	*all or most*	*some or none*	*all or most*	*some or none*
high	43%	32%	39%	27%	52%	39%
medium	23	22	29	33	22	29
low	34	45	32	40	26	32
total per cent	100	100	100	100	100	100
number	(381)	(40)	(185)	(15)	(407)	(31)

source: Rosenberg (1963: 46)

father's side, or identifies with both equally, those who say that their mothers knew few of their friends are less likely to have high self-esteem than those who say she knew many. It is thus questionable whether the original relationship is due to the respondents' dislike of their mothers, since the difference obtains among those who do or do not identify with their mothers in this situation.

But perhaps it is not the respondent's *present* identification with the mother, but his past reactions to her, which are crucial. In other words, the adolescent may remember disliking his mother when he was ten or eleven and may thus assume that she knew nothing of his friends at that time. In order to examine this point, respondents were asked, 'When you were about ten or eleven years old, to whom were you most likely to talk about personal things?' *Table 9* shows that whether the child said he confided mostly in his mother, in some other person, or

Table 9   *Reports of mother's knowledge of child's friends and subject's self-esteem, by tendency to confide in others*

	most likely to talk about personal things to ...					
	mother		other person		no one or can't remember	
	mother knew friends ...					
respondent's self-esteem	all or most	some or none	all or most	some or none	all or most	some or none
high	51%	39%	41%	35%	46%	29%
medium	23	32	26	20	21	30
low	26	29	33	45	34	41
total per cent	100	100	100	100	100	100
number	(540)	(41)	(537)	(55)	(195)	(27)

source: Rosenberg (1963: 39)

in no one, those who said their mothers knew most of their friends tended to have higher self-esteem than those who said their mothers knew few of their friends. The result is thus not due to a negative attitude towards the mother during this earlier period under consideration.

But a third possibility must also be considered. It may not be the child's attitude towards his mother in general, but his recollection of how she behaved towards his *friends* in particular, that colors his recollection of whether she knew his friends. If he recalls her as being unpleasant towards his friends, he might assume that she took little interest in knowing who they were. After the adolescents indicated whether their mothers knew most of their friends, they were asked, 'How did she usually act towards them?' *Table 10* (see over) shows that *irrespective of whether the students said their mothers were friendly or not friendly*, those who said their mothers knew most of their friends had higher self-esteem than those who said their mothers knew few of their friends. Their recollection of whether their mothers knew their friends is, then, not

Table 10   *Reports of mother's knowledge of child's friends and subject's self-esteem, by mother's behaviour towards friends*

	how mother acted towards child's friends					
	very friendly		fairly friendly		not friendly	
	mother knew child's friends...					
respondent's self-esteem	all or most	some or none	all or most	some or none	all or most	some or none
high	48%	34%	45%	33%	32%	21%
medium	23	24	26	28	29	26
low	29	41	29	29	40	53
total per cent	100	100	100	100	100	100
number	(1091)	(58)	(259)	(51)	(38)	(19)

source: Rosenberg (1963: 40)

simply a reflection of their favorable or unfavorable memories of their mothers' behavior towards their friends.

We thus see that irrespective of whether the adolescent says he did or did not chiefly confide in his mother at an earlier time; irrespective of whether he identifies with her, with his father, or with both equally at the present time; and irrespective of whether he says she was friendly or unfriendly to his mates, the student who reports that his mother knew most of his friends tends to have higher self-esteem than the one who reports that she knew few. It is likely, then, that the reported differential knowledge of friends does not simply reflect the student's biased perception of, or attitudes towards, the mother.

These three controls, of course, do not firmly establish that the report of mother's knowledge of friends is not contaminated with an associated variable, but they add to one's confidence in the measure. There is now stronger reason to believe that the answers reflect mother's knowledge rather than the biased perception of the respondent.

PART II
Medical education and sociology

5 Does medicine need sociology? A defence of the Todd Commission proposals for broadening the base of medical education

Margot Jefferys*

[*This paper is complete. The author is Professor of Medical Sociology at Bedford College, University of London, UK.*]

'In parenthesis, it has been a source of pleasure to some of us lewd fellows of the baser sort to note the lack of enthusiasm at QMC for instituting the dreaded department of sociology as part of the price it must pay for acquiring a medical faculty.'

So wrote Professor Warren, who holds the Chair of Biochemistry at the London Hospital Medical College, in the University of London *Bulletin* (Warren 1973). He may or may not be right in suggesting that Queen Mary College dreads the advent of a sociology department; but because he has confessed to some pleasure at QMC's discomfort, I have taken it that Professor Warren himself is not particularly enamoured of sociology and is not keen to see it as a integral part of the medical education, to which he himself contributes an essential ingredient. Since he may not be alone in holding this opinion, and since it is one which I believe is ultimately detrimental to the interests of the consumers of

*from the University of London *Bulletin* (1974) (6): 7–9, March

medical services, I have accepted an invitation from the editor of the *Bulletin* to respond to this comment.

Up to the present, the main emphasis in medical education has been on training people to deal with pathological conditions which cut human life short or cause pain. There is an increasing body of knowledge about these conditions, why they occur, how they can be diagnosed, who is most susceptible to them, and how they can be prevented or reversed. This knowledge comes predominantly from laboratory research backed by clinical trials and epidemiological enquiry. Students must therefore know something of the sciences on which they are based. There is too great a body of knowledge for any single doctor to be expert over the whole range, but there is a modicum which all of them must learn. Briefly, this is the rationale for the shape of the present day medical curriculum.

In the meantime, however, in the most prosperous countries, the changing pattern of health and disease has meant that medicine is now called upon to deal mainly with conditions which are not life-threatening emergencies, but which prevent individuals from performing self-supportive activities, from developing intellectual and physical potentials, and from achieving an inner sense of well-being. While no one would argue that doctors should be the only ones to provide services to meet these kinds of need, the public clearly expects them to play a major part in tackling these problems, the solutions to which present just as much of a challenge as any the medical scientist now faces. The question is whether he should confine his role to that of mastering and applying the knowledge which is a spin-off from his traditional concern with organic pathology or whether he should also attempt to master the behavioural sciences which will undoubtedly provide the main clues to understanding the psychopathology and social pathology inherent in the aetiology of the condition as well as its course once it is under treatment.

Let us assume for a moment that the doctor is only to be concerned with organic pathology and is prepared to allow other non-medically qualified professional workers such as clinical psychologists and social workers to take the main responsibility for the diagnosis and treatment of non-organic illness. If this were to be the case, doctors would need to work in egalitarian harness with other professional groups. The fine demarcation between what is organic and what psychopathological is hardly appreciated by the mass of uninitiated patients whose physical lesions may only lead them to seek care because they are emotionally distressed and socially embarrassed by them. But supposing doctors were to insist that their role was to be confined to treating the physical lesions, they would still need to acquire enough understanding of human behaviour and how it is sustained or altered by pressures from the social environment to enable them to work effectively in a team with those who were experts in psychological and social pathology. They would still need to know how to treat their patients with dignity and understanding.

Many doctors will claim that they already acquire such knowledge and skills during their medical apprenticeship, not by formal teaching in the behavioural sciences, but by experimentation and experience and by observing their medical preceptors at work. There is enough evidence, however, to suggest that the absence of theory and the haphazard way in which interpersonal skills are acquired accounts for the learning, if it occurs at all, being unnecessarily long, drawn out, and less effective in practice than it could be. Studies of patients in the United States and in Britain, for example, have demonstrated that doctors frequently fail to extract relevant information from their patients or to treat them with empathy with the result that their service is not as effective as it could be. Other studies have also suggested that failure to understand the social pressures to which they and other health professionals are subjected results in dysfunctional frustration among doctors and wastage among nursing students. In short, the evidence of poor doctor performance in interpersonal relationships is sufficiently strong to suggest that it is worth introducing medical students systematically to some of the more relevant concepts in the behavioural sciences.

If we accept the much more realistic assumption that the doctor is not likely to confine his role in the treatment of diseases entirely to their organic manifestations, then we must insist that he become aware of the way in which man's social environment, interacting with his genetically determined constitution, contributes to particular pathological states and to his response to attempts to reverse or control these states. Evidence is accumulating, indeed, that man's social environment is a component in the aetiology of nearly all the diseases which doctors are called upon to deal with and that the outcome of treatment depends equally upon how favourable that social environment is. Hence, even the surgeon who is called upon to make decisions about a kidney transplant should be able to perform a more valuable social role if he has some knowledge of the ways in which man's social relationships influence his health state and his health behaviour. At the other extreme of the spectrum of medical specialties, the general practitioner (and more than one-half of all our medical graduates are needed in general practice) will be particularly severely handicapped if he does not possess such knowledge. So, too, will our future psychiatrists, geriatricians, and other specialists who are in particularly short supply given the changes in our demographic structure and disease patterns.

In theory, the wider society has possessed the right since the formation of the General Medical Council in 1858 to take part in the decisions as to the kind of education which will best fit the men and women who choose and are chosen for a medical career to be 'safe' doctors. Moreover, at least in Britain, since 1948, most doctors receive their education largely at public expense. Any early sacrifice which they or their parents make while they receive it is more than amply rewarded by their later earning capacity, by the esteem in which they are held by their countrymen, and by their opportunity for intrinsically rewarding work. They work either in publicly provided hospital facilities or, if they are general practitioners, derive most of their income direct from the national coffers.

In practice, the decisions as to what should be taught have been left largely to the comparatively small consortia of clinicians, biochemists, physiologists, and anatomists who form self-perpetuating oligarchies in the medical schools. It is they who interpret the general regulations laid down decennially by the GMC. The willingness to leave it to the profession could be regarded as a demonstration of faith in the profession's disinterested concern for its patients, and it is true that the profession does enjoy such a reputation among the vast majority of the population; moreover, since much of the knowledge the profession acquires is esoteric, it can be properly argued that the public is best served by leaving considerations of the content of medical education to the experts.

The absence of outside interference with the profession's conduct of the education of its neophytes or with its standards of practice more generally could, however, be held to have been partly responsible for the production of doctors who are qualified, neither intellectually nor emotionally, to make as significant a contribution to the problems which are presented to them as they should be. While medical students acquire technological skills as well as an esoteric knowledge of cellular structure and a variety of pathological agents which may attack it, they are often woefully ignorant of the psychosocial factors which are implicated both in their patients' somatic symptoms and in their response to treatment. However good they may be as technologists, they are ill-equipped to act as applied behavioural scientists, an approach which is required if they are to be entitled to their claim to take a holistic view of their healing functions.

Moreover, the medical schools turn out too many individuals who want to be consultant physicians and surgeons or super-specialists and too few who want to be general practitioners and psychiatrists. The London medical schools are the worst offenders in this respect. Indeed, I have sometimes had the impression that they count their successes in terms of the size of the proportion of their students who go on to become consultants in specialist medicine, the bigger the better. They appear to agree with Lord Moran's reported statement that the man who enters general practice has 'fallen off the ladder of success'. It is in pursuit of this cause, presumably, that medical students spend hours learning by rote facts which they do not retain much beyond their second MB examinations, and which would in any case be of little use even if they were able to retain them. Equally depressing is the fact that far too many students acquire, along with the soon-to-be-forgotten facts, a rigidity of mind and a diminution of curiosity about the human condition itself.

Fortunately, a substantial proportion of medical students are intelligent enough to withstand the pressures of this cloying environment. It is they who are asking that they should not be cut off from the serious study of the society in which they will work and its effects upon the men, women, and children who will be their patients, and on themselves. They are supported by an increasing number of general practitioners who feel they were cheated by the narrowness of their own medical training and want the next generation of doctors to be better equipped than they felt they were when they emerged from medical schools and hospital-based house jobs to face the realities of medicine outside the hospital walls.

In the sense that sociology does not take the claims of professions at their face value but examines them for their social implications, it can of course be disturbing. Those who learn to think in sociological terms, for example, are apt to ask questions which may be embarrassing for those who have become accustomed to unquestioning obedience. Back in the 1830s, Brunel the engineer, giving evidence to a committee concerned with the education of the working classes, argued that he would not want his engineers to be able to read, because it would distract them from their specific function, locomotive driving. Perhaps it did. Perhaps we would not have experienced the inconvenience of the train drivers' recent work-to-rule if they had not been able to read. The spread of literacy has certainly been one factor in the continuing redistribution of power and economic rewards which has since taken place and will continue to take place. The spread of sociology may well be a further influence on that distribution and the future. On the other hand, it can be as intellectually exciting and helpful to the medical profession as it prepares to meet tomorrow's challenges as literacy proved to be for generations of working people. I hope Professor Warren and his colleagues, so far from 'dreading' its advent, will seek to provide optimum conditions for its incorporation in the education of students for whom they are responsible.

6 History-taking for medical students: deficiencies in performance

Peter Maguire &
*Derek R. Rutter**

[*This paper is complete. The authors are a psychiatrist and psychologist, respectively, working in the UK.*]

Introduction

The initial history is a fundamental aspect of clinical practice (Hampton, *et al.* 1975). It is, therefore, essential that doctors are equipped with the skills required to elicit information that is both accurate and relevant to an understanding of their patients' problems. It is also crucial that they learn to establish effective relationships with their patients. However, studies that have monitored directly the performances of medical students with general medical and surgical patients, suggest that students lack basic history-taking skills (Anderson, *et al.* 1970; Tapia, 1972). These deficiencies include an inability to keep patients to the point and to clarify the real nature of patients' complaints, reluctance to ask about relevant psychological and social aspects of their histories, and failure to pick up important verbal and non-verbal cues.

These studies have been carried out with inexperienced students, and

* extracted from The *Lancet* (1976): 556–58, September 11

it is possible to argue that their further clinical training makes good these deficiencies. However, given the nature of the difficulties and the methods traditionally used to teach history-taking, we considered it much more likely that such improvements do not occur. We hypothesized, therefore, that senior medical students would display the same deficiencies in their history-taking skills. We sought to test this by a detailed analysis of histories conducted by a series of senior medical students.

Methods

Fifty medical students at the University of Oxford who were doing a clerkship in psychiatry were consecutively included, provided that they were within fifteen months of their final examinations and had completed firms in medicine, surgery, paediatrics, and obstetrics and gynaecology. The students were each asked to interview a psychiatric patient previously unknown to them. They were told that they had fifteen minutes to determine the patient's present problems and that it was their responsibility to end their interviews on time. Students were also informed that the purpose of the exercise was to assess their history-taking skills, and that they should write up a careful history afterwards. Finally, they were given their patients' names and told that they should assume that their patients were ignorant about the task in hand.

The exercise was designed to test basic history-taking skills only. Patients were, therefore, selected as follows: they were recovering from a depressive illness or anxiety state, were very willing to cooperate, and were able to give a good and coherent history within the time. Each interview was recorded on videotape. The recordings were then analyzed to find out the extent to which the students displayed skills in history-taking. This was done by means of a rating scale specially developed for the purpose (Maguire, Clarke, and Jolly unpublished).

Where the technique was discrete, such as a student explaining who he was, it was simply rated as present (1) or absent (0). When the technique was complex, for example 'helping the patient keep to the point', a five-point scale from 0-4 was used. A score of 0 meant that the student was 'very poor', allowing the patient to spend all the time talking of matters quite irrelevant to the task in hand. A score of 4 meant that the student encouraged the patient to be relevant throughout the interview and so was rated as 'very good'. The written histories were analyzed in terms of the number of items of accurate and relevant information which they contained. Judgements of relevance were based on the patient's case-notes.

Results

Amount of data elicited

It was particularly worrying to find that 24 per cent of the students failed to discover their patients' main problems. In all, the students reported a median of only fourteen items of information in their histories. This represented just one-third of the data which were readily obtainable in the time allowed. The students reported virtually no data about the effects the psychiatric illness had had on their patients' marriages, sexual adjustment, or day-to-day functioning, or about what supports, if any, they had had. When these results were fed back to the students they were surprised; they had all considered themselves very much more efficient at gathering information.

Deficiencies in technique

When beginning their interviews, most students (78 per cent) gave clear greetings to the patients and addressed them by their correct names (88 per cent). Slightly fewer (70 per cent) indicated verbally or by gesture where the patients should sit. Although they were meeting these patients for the first time, 30 per cent of students did not introduce themselves by name, 44 per cent failed to mention they were medical students, and 68 per cent neglected to explain the firms to which they were attached. Only 16 per cent of students bothered to check that their patients understood that the interviews were being recorded and filmed and that this was acceptable. Even fewer students (4 per cent) gave any indication of the time they had or the fact that they would like to take notes, or checked that the patient was at ease. Only 8 per cent explained the purpose of their interviews.

The students were rated on ten items for their performance in taking the main history, and the results are shown in *Table 11* (see over).

(1) *Avoidance of more personal issues.* 36 per cent of students avoided asking any specific questions or responding to any cues about their patients' personal relationships, sexual adjustment, or feelings about their illnesses. They also neglected to check whether or not their patients had felt suicidal. A further 44 per cent touched on these matters only very superficially, even though their patients had volunteered them as problems.

(2) *Acceptance of jargon.* When patients used phrases such as 'feeling run down', 'depressed', or 'tense' to describe their complaints, only 8 per cent of students attempted routinely to

Table 11   *Ratings of history-taking techniques*

techniques used	poor or very poor (0 or 1)	neither good nor poor (2)	good or very good (3 or 4)
coverage of more personal topics	40 (80%)	9 (18%)	1 (2%)
acceptance of jargon	39 (78%)	7 (14%)	4 (8%)
precision	43 (86%)	6 (12%)	1 (2%)
picking up verbal leads	37 (74%)	11 (22%)	2 (4%)
repetition of topics	36 (72%)	14 (28%)	0 (0%)
clarification	31 (62%)	15 (30%)	4 (8%)
control	27 (54%)	18 (36%)	5 (10%)
facilitation	16 (32%)	27 (54%)	7 (14%)
use of leading questions	17 (34%)	29 (58%)	5 (10%)
use of complex questions	12 (24%)	21 (42%)	17 (34%)

establish what they really meant. Seventy-eight per cent of students simply took such statements at face value. In consequence several of them were seriously misled about the true nature of their patients' problems.

(3) *Imprecision.* The majority of students (86 per cent) made little effort to date the key events in their patients' histories precisely or to determine the names, duration, dosages, and effects of any treatments which had been prescribed.

(4) *Failure to pick up verbal leads.* All the patients provided many useful verbal cues about the nature of their problems. Hence it was disconcerting that 74 per cent of the students failed to pick up more than a fraction of these. Only 4 per cent of students were able consistently to detect and use the cues given to them. Patients were often forced to repeat key phrases such as 'I was feeling very low' as many as ten times in order to try to get the students to acknowledge their mood disturbance.

(5) *Repetition.* It would be some comfort if the low amount of information obtained could be attributed to the time limits imposed. However, this claim is difficult to sustain given the finding that 72 per cent of students lost much time through needlessly repeating topics already well covered.

(6) *Lack of clarification.* 62 per cent of students failed to confront patients with the marked inconsistencies or gaps in their stories. The information elicited was frequently confused and conflicting. Only 8 per cent obtained a 'good' or 'very good' rating on this item.

(7) *Lack of control.* Over half the students (54 per cent) allowed their patients to talk about irrelevant matters without making any but the most hesitant attempts to interrupt them and bring them back to the point. Yet where five other students made consistent attempts to keep their patients to the point the patients were eager to cooperate.

(8) *Facilitation.* The students experienced much less difficulty in encouraging their patients to talk. Even so, 32 per cent gave little or no indication that they wanted their patients to continue talking. Instead, they often buried their heads in their notes and rarely, if ever, looked at their patients.

(9) *Inappropriate question style.* Thirty-four per cent of students put questions in a form which led their patients to answer in a particular way. For example, they would ask, 'you were waking up early?' rather than, 'did you notice any change in your sleeping habits?'. Twenty-four per cent made their questions so complicated and lengthy that it was impossible for the patients to recall the separate elements or give appropriate answers.

(10) *Other difficulties.* We noted that most students assumed that there would only be one illness or problem. They usually seized on the first complaint volunteered and did not bother to check whether there could be others of equal or greater importance. They then adopted a mode of history-taking oriented either to physical or to psychiatric illness. They did not seem able to cope with the possibility that both might be present. Whichever scheme they followed, they found it difficult to tailor it to the task they had been given.

Only 10 per cent of the students ended their interviews in the time. Even fewer (8 per cent) attempted to check that they had got the history right before they finished.

Discussion

Our analysis revealed serious deficiencies in the history-taking skills of these senior medical students, and confirmed that the deficiencies are identical to those found in less experienced medical students. However, since these deficiencies were revealed in a test situation, it could be argued that they represent a response to our particular task rather than the students' true history-taking abilities.

We arranged, therefore, for audiotape recordings to be made of twelve of these students while they were taking histories from new out-patients. Comparison of these histories with those taken in the test showed identical deficiencies in technique. We thus think it reasonable to conclude that these deficiencies are real, particularly as the students readily acknowledged them.

Support for this view comes from the work of Helfer. He found that senior medical students were much more likely than inexperienced students to ask leading questions, avoid emotional aspects of cases, use medical jargon, and ignore important cues. Furthermore, when medical students are asked what difficulties they have when talking to patients they describe exactly similar problems to those we found (MacNamara 1974). If our findings are valid, similar deficiencies should be evident in qualified doctors who have received the same type of training. Studies of the practice of physicians (Maguire, et al. 1974), paediatricians (Korsch, et al. 1968), surgeons (Maguire 1976), and general practitioners (Goldberg and Blackwell 1970) confirm this.

While the nature and magnitude of these deficiencies may be depressing, they should not be surprising. Little time is yet devoted in most medical school curricula to formal training in history-taking skills. The time that is given is usually taken up with a few seminars and demonstrations which focus on the questions which should be asked to elicit physical illness. Little guidance is given about the techniques which should be used or about coverage of the psychological and social aspects of each case. Thereafter, a student's learning is generally based on his tutor's appraisal of the histories when he reports back in seminars or on ward rounds. Little attention is likely to be paid to how the student obtained his data or related to his patient. It is also most unlikely that the tutor will have actually observed his student taking a history.

A further problem arises from the history-taking schemes which the student is given by various departments. These are likely to be fragmented and conflicting, and so make it difficult for the student to develop the holistic approach which he will need to adopt if he is to meet the needs of his patients and overcome the constraints of limited time which he will meet in real practice.

It seems probable, therefore, that the history-taking skills of medical students could be much improved if these gaps in training were remedied. We suggest that this could be done as follows: by giving students a more detailed and relevant model of how to take an initial history and what questions to ask; by giving them a chance to practise this under conditions of direct observation within strict time limits; and by providing them with feedback about their performance.

Indeed, we have already put these suggestions to the test, and, as we report in another paper (Rutter and Maguire 1976) and in a recent review, (Maguire and Rutter 1976b) the results have been encouraging. They indicate that much could be done of a practical nature to help medical students and doctors to improve their history-taking skills, particularly if such training were given at the beginning of their clinical course, or even pre-clinically (*British Medical Journal* 1976).

PART III
The family, marriage, and its relationship to illness

7 The psychological meaning of mental illness in the family

Marian Radke-Yarrow, Charlotte Green Schwarz, Harriet S. Murphy, &
*Leila Calhoun Deasy**

[*This paper has been edited from the original mainly by the deletion of a very informative, but very long, case history. The authors are now chief of a laboratory of developmental psychology, a clinical sociologist, a social psychologist, and a Professor of social work, respectively, in the USA.*]

This paper presents an analysis of cognitive and emotional problems encountered by the wife in coping with the mental illness of her husband. It is concerned with the factors which lead to the reorganization of the wife's perceptions of her husband from a *well* man to a man who is mentally sick or in need of hospitalization in a mental hospital.

Ideally, to study this problem one might like to interview the wives as they struggled with the developing illness. This is precluded, however, by the fact that the problem is not 'visible' until psychiatric help is sought. The data, therefore, are the wives' reconstructions of their earlier experiences and accounts of their current reactions during the husband's hospitalization.

It is recognized that recollections of the prehospital period may well include systematic biases, such as distortions, omissions, and increased organization and clarity. As a reliability check, a number of wives, just before the husband's discharge from the hospital, were asked again

*extracted from The Journal of Social Issues (1955) II: 12–24

to describe the events and feelings of the prehospital period. In general, the two reports are markedly similar; often details are added and others are elaborated, but events tend to be substantially the same. While this check attests to the consistency of the wives' reporting, it has, of course, the contamination of over-learning which comes from many retellings of these events.

Our analysis is concerned primarily with the process of the wife's getting to this stage in interpreting and responding to the husband's behavior. Some general trends appear in the data. These trends can be systematized in terms of the following focal aspects of the process:

1 The wife's threshold for initially discerning a problem depends on the accumulation of various kinds of behavior which are not readily understandable or acceptable to her.

2 This accumulation forces upon the wife the necessity for examining and adjusting expectations for herself and her husband which permit her to account for his behavior.

3 The wife is in an 'overlapping' situation, of problem – not problem, of normal – not normal. Her interpretations shift back and forth.

4 Adaptations to the atypical behavior of the husband occur. There is testing and waiting for additional cues in coming to any given interpretation, as in most problem solving. The wife mobilizes strong defenses against the husband's deviant behavior. These defenses take form in such reactions as denying, attenuating, balancing, and normalizing the husband's problems.

5 Eventually there is a threshold point at which the perception breaks, when the wife comes to the relatively stable conclusion that the problem is a psychiatric one and/or that she cannot alone cope with the husband's behavior.

These processes are elaborated in the following analysis of the wives' responses.

The beginnings of the wife's concern

In the early interviews, the wife was asked to describe the beginnings of the problem which led to her husband's hospitalization. ('Could you tell me when you first noticed that your husband was different?') This question was intended to provide an orientation for the wife to reconstruct the sequence and details of events and feelings which characterized the period preceding hospitalization. The interviewer provided a minimum of structuring in order that the wife's emphases and organization could be obtained.

In retrospect, the wives usually cannot pinpoint the time the husband's problem emerged. Neither can they clearly carve it out from the contexts of the husband's personality and family expectations. The subjective beginnings are seldom localized in a single strange or disturbing reaction on the husband's part but rather in the piling up of behavior and feelings. Thus, Mrs Q. verbalizes the impact of a concentration of changes which occur within a period of a few weeks. Her explicit recognition of a problem comes when she adds up this array; her husband stays out late, doesn't eat or sleep, has obscene thoughts, argues with her, hits her, talks continuously, 'cannot appreciate the beautiful scene', and 'cannot appreciate me or the baby'.

The problem behaviors reported by the wives are given in *Table 12* (see over). They are ordered roughly; the behaviors listed first occurred primarily, but not exclusively, within the family; those later occurred in the more public domain. Whether the behavior is public or private does not seem to be a very significant factor in determining the wife's threshold for perceiving a problem.

There are many indications that these behaviors, now organized as a problem, have occurred many times before. This is especially true where alcoholism, physical complaints, or personality 'weaknesses' enter the picture. The wives indicate how, earlier, they had assimilated these characteristics into their own expectations in a variety of ways: the characteristics were congruent with their image of their husbands, they fitted their differential standards for men and women (men being less able to stand up to troubles), they had social or environmental justifications, etc.

When and how behavior becomes defined as problematic appears to be a highly individual matter. In some instances, it is when the wife can no longer manage her husband (he will no longer respond to her usual prods); in others, when his behavior destroys the *status quo* (when her goals and living routines are disorganized); and, in still others, when she cannot explain his behavior.

Initial interpretations of husband's problem

Once the behavior is organized as a problem, it tends also to be interpreted as some particular kind of problem. More often than not, however, the husband's difficulties are not seen initially as manifestations of mental illness or even as emotional problems (*Table 13* see over).

Early interpretations often tend to be organized around physical

Table 12   *Reported problem behavior at time of the wife's initial concern and at time of the husband's admission to hospital*

	initially		at hospital admission	
problem behavior	psychotics N	psycho-neurotics N	psychotics N	psycho-neurotics N
physical problems, complaints, worries	12	5	7	5
deviations from routines of behavior	17	9	13	9
expressions of inadequacy or hopelessness	4	1	5	2
nervous, irritable, worried	19	10	18	9
withdrawal (verbal, physical)	5	1	6	1
changes or accentuations in personality 'traits' (slovenly, deceptive, forgetful)	5	6	7	6
aggressive or assaultive and suicidal behavior	6	3	10	6
strange or bizarre thoughts, delusions, hallucinations, and strange behavior	11	1	15	2
excessive drinking	4	7	3	4
violation of codes of 'decency'	3	1	3	2
number of respondents	23	10	23	10

Table 13   *Initial interpretations of the husband's behaviour*

interpretation	psychotics N	psychoneurotics N
nothing really wrong	3	0
'character' weakness and 'controllable' behavior (lazy, mean, etc.)	6	3
physical problem	6	0
normal response to crisis	3	1
mildly emotionally disturbed	1	2
'something' seriously wrong	2	2
serious emotional or mental problem	2	2
number of respondents	23	10

difficulties (18 per cent of cases) or 'character' problems (27 per cent). For example, Mrs Y., whose husband was chronically alcoholic, aggressive, and threatening to her, 'raving', and who 'chewed his nails until they almost bled', interprets his difficulty thus: 'He was just spoiled rotten. He never outgrew it. He told me when he was a child he could get his own way if he insisted, and he is still that way.' This quotation is the prototype of many of its kind.

Some wives, on the other hand, locate the problem in the environment. They expect the husband to change as the environmental crisis subsides.

Where the wives interpret the husband's difficulty as emotional in nature, they tend to be inconsistently 'judgmental' and 'understanding'. The psychoneurotics are more often perceived initially by their wives as having emotional problems or as being mentally ill than are the psychotics. This is true even though many more clinical signs (bizarre, confused, delusional, aggressive, and disoriented behavior) are reported by the wives of the psychotics than of the psychoneurotics.

Initial interpretations, whatever their content, are seldom held with great confidence by the wives. Many recall their early reactions to their husbands' behaviors as full of puzzling confusion and uncertainty. Something is wrong, they know, but, in general, they stop short of a firm explanation. Thus, Mrs M. reports, 'He was kind of worried. He was kind of worried before, not exactly worried...' She thought of his many physical complaints; she 'racked' her 'brain' and told her husband, 'Of course he didn't feel good'. Finally, he stayed home from work with 'no special complaints, just blah', and she 'began to realize it was more deeply seated'.

Changing perceptions of the husband's problem

The fog and uneasiness in the wife's early attempts to understand and cope with the husband's difficulties are followed, typically, by painful psychological struggles to resolve the uncertainties and to change the current situation. Usually, the wife's perceptions of the husband's problems undergo a series of changes before hospitalization is sought or effected, irrespective of the length of time elapsing between the beginnings of concern and hospitalization.

Viewing these changes macroscopically, three relatively distinct patterns of successive redefinitions of the husband's problems are apparent. One sequence is characterized by a progressive intensification; interpretations are altered in a definite direction – towards seeing the problem as mental illness. Mrs O. illustrates this progression. Initially, she thought her husband was 'unsure of himself'. 'He was worried,

too, about getting old.' These ideas moved to: 'He'd drink to forget
... He just didn't have the confidence ... He'd forget little things ...
He'd wear a suit weeks on end if I didn't take it away from him ...
He'd say nasty things.' Then, when Mr O. seemed 'so confused', 'to
forget all kinds of things ... where he'd come from ... to go to work',
and made 'nasty, cutting remarks all the time', she began to think
in terms of a serious personality disturbance. 'I did think he knew that
something was wrong ... that he was sick. He was never any different
this last while and I couldn't stand it any more ... You don't know
what a relief it was...' (when he was hospitalized). The husband's
drinking, his failure to be tidy, his nastiness, etc., lose significance in
their own right. They move from emphasis to relief and are recast as
signs of 'something deeper', something that brought 'it' on.

Some wives whose interpretations move in the direction of seeing
their husbands as mentally ill hold conceptions of mental illness and of
personality that do not permit assigning the husband all aspects of the
sick role. Frequently, they use the interpretation of mental illness as
an angry epithet or as a threatening prediction for the husband. This
is exemplified in such references as: 'I told him he should have his
head examined', 'I called him a half-wit', 'I told him if he's not
careful, he'll be a mental case'. To many of these wives, the hospital
is regarded as the 'end of the road'.

A somewhat different pattern of sequential changes in interpreting
the husband's difficulties is to be found among wives who appear to cast
around for situationally and momentarily adequate explanations. As the
situation changes or as the husband's behavior changes, these wives find
reasons and excuses but lack an underlying or synthesizing theory. Successive interpretations tend to bear little relation to one another. Situational
factors tend to lead them to seeing their husbands as mentally ill. Immediate, serious, and direct physical threats or the influence of others
may be the deciding factor. For example, a friend or employer may insist
that the husband see a psychiatrist, and the wife goes along with the
decision.

A third pattern of successive redefinitions revolves around an orientation outside the framework of emotional problems or mental illness. In
these cases, the wife's specific explanations change but pivot around a
denial that the husband is mentally ill.

A few wives seem not to change their interpretations about their
husband's difficulties. They maintain the same explanation throughout
the development of his illness, some within the psychiatric framework,
others rigidly outside that framework.

The process of recognizing the husband's problem as mental illness

In the total situation confronting the wife, there are a number of factors, apparent in our data, which make it difficult for the wife to recognize and accept the husband's behavior in a mental-emotional-psychiatric framework. Many cross-currents seem to influence the process.

The husband's behavior itself is a fluctuating stimulus. He is not worried and complaining all of the time. His delusions and hallucinations may not persist.

The relationship between husband and wife also supplies a variety of images and contexts which can justify varied conclusions about the husband's current behavior. The wife is likely to adapt to behavior which occurs in their day-to-day relationships. Therefore, symptomatic reactions which are intensifications of long-standing response patterns become part of the fabric of life and are not easily disentangled as 'symptomatic'.

The larger social context contributes, too, in the wife's perceptual tug of war. Others with whom she can compare her husband provide contrasts to his deviance, but others (Mr F.'s nervous friends) also provide parallels to his problems. The 'outsiders', seeing less of her husband, often discount the wife's alarm when she presses them for opinions. In other instances, the friend or employer, less adapted to or defended against the husband's symptoms, helps her to define his problem as psychiatric.

This task before the wife, of defining her husband's difficulties, can be conceptualized as an 'overlapping' situation (in Lewin's terms), in which the relative potencies of the several effective influences fluctuate. The wife is responding to the various sets of forces simultaneously. Thus, several conclusions or interpretations of the problem are simultaneously 'suspended in balance', and they shift back and forth in emphasis and relief. Seldom, however, does she seem to be balancing off clear-cut alternatives, such as physical versus mental. Her complex perceptions (even those of Mrs F. who is extreme in misperceiving cues) are more 'sophisticated' than the casual questioner might be led to conclude.

Thus far, we have ignored the personally threatening aspects of recognizing mental illness in one's spouse, and the defenses that are mobilized to meet this threat. One or more of the following defenses are manifested in three-fourths of our cases.

The most obvious form of defense in the wife's response is the tendency to *normalize* the husband's neurotic and psychotic symptoms. His behavior is explained, justified, or made acceptable by seeing it also in herself or by assuring herself that the particular behavior occurs again and again among persons who are not ill. Illustrative of this reaction is the wife who reports her husband's hallucinations and assures herself that this is normal because she herself heard voices when she was in the menopause. Another wife responds to her husband's physical complaints, fears, worries, nightmares, and delusions with 'A lot of normal people think there's something wrong when there isn't. I think men are that way; his father is that way.'

When behavior cannot be normalized, it can be made to seem less severe or less important in a total picture than an outsider might see it. By finding some grounds for the behavior or something explainable about it, the wife achieves at least momentary *attenuation* of the seriousness of it. Thus, Mrs F. is able to discount partly the strangeness of her husband's descriptions of the worms growing out of his grandfather's moustache when she recalls his watching the worms in the fish bowl. There may be attenuation, too, by seeing the behavior as 'momentary' ('You could talk him out of his ideas') or by rethinking the problem and seeing it in a different light.

By *balancing* acceptable with unacceptable behavior or 'strange' with 'normal' behavior, some wives can conclude that the husband is not seriously disturbed. Thus, it is very important to Mrs R. that her husband kissed her goodbye before he left for the hospital. This response cancels out his hostile feelings towards her and the possibility that he is mentally ill. Similarly, Mrs V. reasons that her husband cannot be 'out of his mind' for he had reminded her of things she must not forget to do when he went to the hospital.

Defense sometimes amounts to a thorough-going *denial*. This takes the form of denying that the behavior perceived can be interpreted in an emotional or psychiatric framework. In some instances, the wife reports vividly on such behavior as repeated thoughts of suicide, efforts to harm her and the like, and sums it up with 'I thought it was just a whim'. Other wives bend their efforts towards proving the implausibility of mental illness.

After the husband is hospitalized, it might be expected that these denials would decrease to a negligible level. This is not wholly the case, however. Examination of the wives' interpretations just following the husband's admission to the hospital shows that some wives still interpret the husband's behavior in another framework than that of a serious emotional problem or mental illness; some ambivalently and sporadically interpret the behavior as an emotional or mental problem. The majority hold relatively stable interpretations within the framework of a mental problem.

After the husband has been hospitalized for some time, many wives reflect on their earlier tendencies to avoid a definition of mental illness. Such reactions are almost identically described by these wives: 'I put it out of my mind – I didn't want to face it – anything but a mental illness.' 'Maybe I was aware of it. But you know you push things away from you and keep hoping.' 'Now you think maybe you should have known about it. Maybe you should have done more than you did and that worries me.'

There are implications of these findings both for those who are working in the field of prevention of mental illness and early detection of emotional disturbance as well as for the rehabilitation worker. They suggest that to acquaint the public with the nature of mental illness by describing psychotic behaviour and emphasizing its non-threatening aspect is, after all, an intellectualization and not likely to be effective in dealing with the threatening aspects of recognizing mental illness which we have described. Further, it is not enough simply to recognize the fact that the rehabilitation of patients is affected by the attitudes and feelings of the family towards the patient and his illness. Perhaps a better acceptance of the patient can be developed if families who have been unable to deal with the problem of the illness are helped to work through this experience and to deal with their difficulties in accepting the illness and what remains of it after the patient leaves the hospital.

8 The influence of family life on the course of schizophrenic disorders: a replication

*George W. Brown, J. L. T. Birley, & John K. Wing**

[*The lengthy original of this paper is carefully and tightly argued. For consideration of space the editors have followed their general strategy. In particular, a section on psychiatric measurement has been drastically curtailed. The details of the argument and data demonstrating that expressed emotion is an important determinant of outcome independent of many background factors have been omitted. Some clinical implications of the work have also been left out. The authors are Professor of Sociology, the Dean of the Institute of Psychiatry, and Professor of Social Psychiatry, respectively, in the UK.*]

The hypothesis under test is that a high degree of expressed emotion is an index of characteristics in the relatives which are likely to cause a florid relapse of schizophrenic symptoms, independently of other factors such as length of history, type of symptomatology, or severity of previous behaviour disturbance.

Design

The case records were screened of all patients aged eighteen to sixty-four, born in the United Kingdom, and living with relatives at an address in Camberwell in SE London, who were beginning a new period of out-patient or in-patient care at any one of five hospitals serving the area. All those whose records indicated that they might be suffering from schizophrenia were interviewed, using a semi-standardized technique to rate and classify their clinical condition (Wing, *et al.* 1967; Cooper

* extracted from the *British Journal of Psychiatry* (1972) 121: 241–58.

1970; Wing 1970). If a diagnosis of possible or probable schizophrenia was made, the patient was included in the study and further social and clinical information was obtained. To obtain a larger number of patients with recent illnesses, all those with similar characteristics who were admitted to Bexley Hospital and were within five years of their first admission were also included.

In this way, 118 patients were selected but seventeen had to be excluded subsequently for various reasons.

The patients and their families were seen on several occasions by members of the research team (two psychiatrists and three sociologists). Eight types of interview were carried out for each patient and family, and ten if the patient was readmitted in the follow-up period. Two interviews to establish the current mental state of the patient and his social and clinical background were carried out by a research psychiatrist soon after the patient was admitted to hospital. The main family interview was carried out at home by a research sociologist while the patient was still in hospital. It usually took two separate visits to each informant to complete and lasted about three hours in all. A husband or wife was always seen; two parents (or married siblings or pairs of siblings) were interviewed separately by different workers.

Both the current mental state and the family interviews were repeated at the time of follow-up nine months after discharge, and comparable ratings were made. A 'joint interview' about two weeks after discharge was similar to that in an earlier study (Brown, *et al.* 1962). The patient and other members of the family were seen at home for no more than one hour. The interview was concerned with the family's and patient's recent contacts with medical or social services and designed to get everyone talking together on such topics. The scales concerning expressed emotion were completed at the main family interviews and at the joint interview. Patients and family were also seen at any readmission during the nine months after discharge.

Techniques of measurement

1.   *Ratings of emotional response*

The techniques of measuring family variables have been described in detailed elsewhere (Brown and Rutter 1966 (see Reading 1); Rutter and Brown 1966).

(a) *Number of critical comments about someone else in the home.*
Critical comments were judged either by tone of voice or by content

of what was said. For a remark to be judged critical in content there had to be a clear and unambiguous statement of resentment, disapproval, or dislike. Any remark could be rated critical on tone alone, and in making the ratings most emphasis was laid on the interviewer's judgement of tone of voice. The verbal unit of assessment was a statement terminated either by a change of topic or by a question from the interviewer. Only one comment could be counted per unit.

(b) *Hostility*. Hostility was rated as present or absent. It was defined as present if a remark was made indicating the rejection of someone as a person; for example, when someone was criticized for what he was rather than for what he did. Hostility was also regarded as present if critical comments tended to be generalized spontaneously; for example, when one criticism triggered off a string of further criticisms on unrelated topics (e.g., 'He's unhelpful, he's not tidy and in money he's the world's worst').

(c) *Dissatisfaction*. According to our definition, criticism and hostility are based on either negative emotion or a clear statement of resentment, disapproval, dislike, or rejection. Another series of ratings took account of any expression of dissatisfaction, whether or not it warranted inclusion as criticism or hostility. Dissatisfaction was rated on four-point scales describing eight areas of family life. An over-all index was also calculated. Many subjects who were highly dissatisfied were rated low on hostility and criticism; it is possible to be markedly dissatisfied yet express little emotion or resentment.

(d) *Warmth*. This six-point rating was based on the amount of warmth *demonstrated* by the respondent when talking about the particular person in the home. In general, stereotyped endearments were ignored, but positive comments, especially if made spontaneously, were regarded as important. Sympathy and concern, interest in the other as a person, and expressed enjoyment in mutual activities were all relevant. Particular attention was paid to warmth expressed in tone of voice. Negative feelings were deliberately ignored in making the rating, but failure to express warmth in what seemed a relevant situation (for example, when describing the patient's ailments) was taken into account. A judgement was based on the whole interview, but the expression of warmth was most likely to occur in certain sections dealing with leisure, marriage, and communication, and with the patient's behaviour.

(e) *Emotional over-involvement*. This measure was designed to pick up unusually marked concern about the patient. It was rated on the basis either of feelings expressed in the interview itself or of behaviour reported outside it. For example, a top rating on the six-point scale was given when a mother showed obvious and constant anxiety while describing such minor matters as her son's diet and the setting of his alarm clock so that he would wake in time for work. She also showed markedly protective attitudes about her son, who was not obviously handicapped; for example, she said, 'I could go out if I wanted to go out. I don't 'cause I'm looking after Johnny'. The rating was only made in the case of parents, as such over-involvement was very rarely found in interviews with husbands and wives. Although conceptually it is the most complex of the scales, agreement on a specially interviewed series of eighteen parents was 0.90.

The relationship between the scales is much what would be expected. Hostility and criticism are highly related, and warmth is negatively related to criticism and hostility. Emotional over-involvement is positively related to warmth, but only half of those rated as markedly warm also showed marked over-involvement. Finally, emotional over-involvement shows a curvilinear relationship to criticism and hostility: those rated high or low on emotional over-involvement show most criticism or hostility.

(f) *Over-all index of relative's expressed emotion (EE).* Since the total number of patients is small, it is necessary to limit the number of sub-groups produced by each variable. The individual scales were first related to relapse and several methods of combining them into a high expressed emotion (EE) group were explored. All of them produced much the same result. The following indices, in hierarchical order, were finally used to allocate approximately half the families to a high expressed emotion group:

	N (total N observed in brackets)	N added to high EE sub-group
interview with relative		
7+ critical comments	35 (101)	35
marked over-involvement of parents	13 (55)	5
hostility	18 (101)	2
joint interview		
2+ critical comments	9 (62)	1
marked over-involvement of parents	9 (35)	2
hostility	3 (62)	0
		45

The joint interview was considerably shorter than that with the relative alone, and rather less emotion was expressed, the relative presumably being more restrained in the presence of the patient. Only three additional cases were added to the group by using the data from the joint interview. Even this small number was only reached by considerably lowering the threshold of definition (to two critical comments, and a score of 2 on the scale of emotional over-involvement). Only one of the three additional patients relapsed.

2   *Measures of behaviour before and at the time of admission*

Many measures of the patient's behaviour before admission were employed in the study. Some of the most important are:

> (i) *Work impairment.* Unemployment or, for housewives, marked handicap in carrying out domestic duties, for at least three months out of the preceding two years. Time in hospital was not taken into account.
>
> (ii) *Disturbed behaviour.* Definite aggressive or delinquent behaviour in the twelve months before admission (forty patients) or very markedly disturbed behaviour at about the time of admission (this added seven patients).
>
> (iii) *Social withdrawal.* A score based on (a) contacts with friends; (b) casual contacts outside the home; (c) contacts within the home.

3   *Psychiatric measures*

All patients were interviewed using the semi-standardized 'Present State Examination', with the main object of describing fairly precisely the symptomatic condition of those included (Wing, *et al.* 1967). The CATEGO clinical classification procedure (Wing, Cooper, and Sartorius 1974) was then applied. Three groups of patients, with the following characteristics, were finally set up:

> (i) Definite schizophrenia ($N = 51$).
>
> (ii) Possible schizophrenia ($N = 42$).
>
> (iii) Doubtful schizophrenia ($N = 8$).

4   Relapse

We distinguished between two types of relapse: type I involved a change from a 'normal' or 'non-schizophrenic' state to a state of 'schizophrenia' as defined in the previous section. Type II involved a marked exacerbation of persistent schizophrenic symptoms. At our interviews at follow-up or readmission, we made a judgement, based on all available information, on two points: first, whether the patient had experienced schizophrenic symptoms at some time during the follow-up period; and second, whether those patients who had been continuously ill had experienced a marked exacerbation of these symptoms.

Table 14 shows the relationships between relapse, symptoms, and readmission of the thirty-five patients who had relapsed during the follow-up period. Twenty-nine of the thirty-five were readmitted. The remaining six all had schizophrenic symptoms at their follow-up interview; five of these patients had been well for some time after their key discharge, while the sixth had been continuously ill and had experienced a marked exacerbation of symptoms shortly before interview.

Three of the readmitted patients had not relapsed. Seventeen of the

Table 14   *Relapse, symptomatology, and readmission*

	readmitted	not readmitted	total
relapse ($N = 35$)			
type I	18	5	23
type II	11	1	12
no relapse ($N = 66$)			
no schizophrenic symptoms	3	46	49
schizophrenic symptoms +	0	17	17
total	32	69	101

the 'not relapsed' patients had experienced schizophrenic symptoms continuously during the follow-up period, but these symptoms had remained steady or showed only mild fluctuations.

5   Time relationships between variables

The indices of work impairment and disturbed behaviour relate to events that are past by the time the patient is admitted to hospital. The scales of expressed emotion are rated while the patient is still in hospital or shortly after discharge. The index of symptomatic relapse relates to events during the year after discharge.

We are making the assumption, therefore, that a high degree of expressed emotion on one occasion is a measure of the relative's propensity to react in that way to that particular patient, even though other factors may be needed to precipitate this. The same relative would not necessarily respond to other people in the same way. For example, there is very little correlation between the amount of emotion expressed by a parent towards the patient and the amount of emotion expressed by the same parent towards his or her spouse. The measure reflects a quality of relationship with a particular person (the patient), not a general tendency to react to everyone in a similar way.

Thus the level of expressed emotion at the time of the patient's key admission will be taken to represent an enduring potential characteristic of the relative's behaviour towards the patient.

Results

Relationship between index of expressed emotion and relapse

The proportions of patients with relatives in the high and low EE groups who relapsed are shown in *Table 15*. There is a significant association between high EE and relapse ($\gamma = 0.75$, 1 df, $p < 0.001$).

Table 15 *Relationship of relatives' emotion to relapse in the 9 months after discharge*

EE of relatives	no relapse	relapse	% relapse
high	19	26	58
low	47	9	16

This result is confirmed when various other indices of high expressed emotion are examined. Measures of critical comments, hostility, or emotional over-involvement of the parents are all significantly associated with relapse.

The other major affective variable measured was dissatisfaction. There was an over-all association between dissatisfaction on the part of relatives and the patient's relapse, but only within the high EE group. This suggests that dissatisfaction as such did not cause relapse.

Ratings of expressed emotion in the patients showed far less than in relatives (only 10 per cent of patients were markedly critical about relatives at home compared with 34 per cent of relatives about patients) and there was no relationship to relapse.

The effect of previous behavioural and work impairment

Work impairment during the two years before key admission was related to relapse ($\gamma = 0.40$), as was disturbed behaviour ($\gamma = 0.32$). An index combining these two factors did not much increase the association ($\gamma = 0.47$). Both were closely related to EE (work impairment, $\gamma = 0.73$; behavioural disturbance, $\gamma = 0.82$). Two-thirds of patients who had been disturbed or had had work difficulties lived with a relative with a high level of EE, but only 14 per cent without such behaviour did so.

There are two alternative ways of explaining this set of correlations. The first and most straightforward hypothesis is that past impairments and disturbances are predictive of future behaviour such as relapse because some underlying 'process' links them together. At the same time, the more disturbed the patient's behaviour, the more likely are the relatives to respond with criticism, hostility, and emotional over-concern. Thus the correlation between expressed emotion and relapse is spurious in so far as it is mediated by the patient's own behaviour, as shown below:

(A)
$$I/D \begin{array}{l} \nearrow EE \text{ (expressed emotion)} \\ \\ \end{array}$$
$$\text{(impairment/} \searrow R \text{ (relapse)}$$
$$\text{disturbance)}$$

The second hypothesis is that the relatives' expressed emotion contributes to relapse independently of the patient's past behaviour. In other words the patient would be unlikely to relapse, however disturbed or impaired his past behaviour, if there were no 'emotional' tension in the home. The relatives' expressed emotion may be caused by the patient's past behaviour, the emotional expression may have caused the behaviour, or each may have influenced the other; it is impossible to say what is primary in a study of this kind.

The three possibilities may be expressed graphically as follows:

(B_1) $I/D \rightarrow EE \rightarrow R$

(B_2) $EE \begin{array}{l} \nearrow R \\ \searrow I/D \end{array}$

(B_3) $I/D \leftrightarrow EE \rightarrow R$

In each of the cases B_1, B_2, and B_3, it is the relationship between EE and R which can be differentiated from that in case (A).

It is possible to discriminate between these two hypotheses, since if relatives' EE independently contributes to relapse various conditions should hold. (The relevant associations are given in *Figure 4*.)

(i) In the first place when previous work impairment and behavioural disturbance are controlled by standardization the association between EE and relapse should not be much reduced. This is the case (gamma becomes 0.63 instead of 0.75), and these two background factors cannot be producing a spurious effect (Blalock 1960).

(ii) In the second place, since in the three alternatives EE is either an intervening variable (B_1 and B_3) or a common cause of the other factors (B_2), the association between impairment/disturbance and relapse should be greatly decreased when EE is controlled (Blalock 1964). In fact it almost disappears (0.47 to 0.08).

(iii) Finally, it follows from these same considerations that the association between impairment, disturbance, and relapse (0.47) should be weaker than that between impairment/disturbance and EE (0.84) or between EE and relapse (0.75). These conditions also hold.

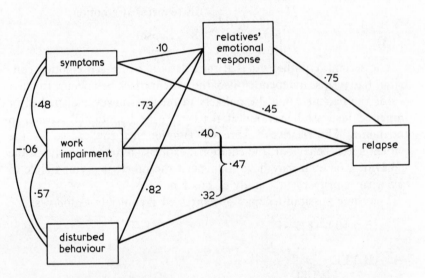

Figure 4   Relationship of the main variables to each other and to relapse.

Clinical picture

Patients who showed 'typical' schizophrenic symptoms (thought intrusion, delusions of control, etc.) at the time of Present State Examination were more likely to relapse than those in the second group ($\gamma = 0.45$). The third (non-paranoid) group is too small for separate analysis and is included with the second.

This association between type of clinical condition and relapse is not mediated by a higher degree of past work impairment or behavioural disturbance (γ for the association between clinical condition and impairment/disturbance is only 0.18; with relapse controlled it is reduced to 0.10). Moreover, the association between EE and relapse remains strong ($\gamma = 0.79$) when type of clinical condition is controlled, and the association between type of clinical condition and relapse is increased slightly ($\gamma = 0.49$) when EE is controlled.

Thus, type of clinical condition is not associated with any particular degree of emotional expression ($\gamma = 0.10$) and seems to be independently related to relapse ($\gamma = 0.49$).

Summary of other factors relating to relapse

Typical schizophrenic symptoms, male sex, acceptance of admission, lack of regular medication, and high contact in the home were associated with a higher chance of relapse. *Table 16* provides a check that the relationship between EE and relapse is not reduced when these factors are controlled. The presence of any such factor scored one point, giving an over-all score from 0 to 5. Relapse is more likely the higher the score, but the association between EE and relapse holds within each score, confirming that it is independent of these factors.

Table 16 *Association between emotional response and relapse controlling for the presence of five factors: type of clinical condition, sex, acceptance or rejection of admission, time in face-to-face contact, and medication*

| | over-all score on five factors | | | | | | | |
| | 5* and 4 | | 3 | | 2 | | 1 and 0* | |
	no relapse	relapse	no relapse	relapse	no relapse	relapse	no relapse	relapse
high EE	1	5	4	16	3	4	10	3
low EE	3	4	14	2	18	1	11	1
γ	0.58		0.93		0.92		0.53	
overall relapse rate as %	69		50		19		16	

*one patient scored 5, and four scored 0

Conclusion and clinical implications

In the first place, the 'emotional involvement' of relatives with patients has been more precisely specified and the term 'expressed emotion' substituted. The most measurable component of expressed emotion is the number of critical comments made by the key relative about the patient. The whole analysis could have been undertaken using this measure alone. However, the other components are important in interpreting the nature of 'expressed emotion'.

Using this index, a high degree of emotion expressed by relatives at the time of key admission was found to be strongly associated with symptomatic relapse during the nine months following discharge. The question arises how far this relationship can be explained by the fact that patients with the most severe behavioural disturbance and work impairment before the time of key admission had the greatest liability to relapse. In our previous study, both factors were independently related to outcome. The present results are unequivocal, however, in suggesting that expressed emotion is independently associated with relapse, while previous work impairment and behavioural disturbance are only associated with relapse because of their association with level of expressed emotion. Moreover, the ability of the index of expressed emotion to predict symptomatic relapse is not explained away by the action of any other factor that we have investigated (such as age, sex, previous occupational record, length of clinical history, type of illness, etc).

The effect of expressed emotion can be mitigated to some extent by two other important environmental variables which might help to give the clinician some control over events. The first of these is regular phenothiazine medication, which shows a close to significant relationship with a favourable outcome. In view of the results obtained in a recent controlled trial of preventive phenothiazine medication (Leff and Wing 1971) this finding must be taken seriously. It is the more significant since, as Leff and Wing found, preventive medication is only effective for certain groups of schizophrenic patients. Our present results suggest that patients living with relatives who expressed high emotion at the time of key admission (and who are therefore most vulnerable to relapse) are also most susceptible to protective drug effects. There is one other clue to the sort of patients most responsive to phenothiazines; those who resisted admission were particularly likely to be living with relatives who expressed high emotion, and they were particularly helped by drugs. The second mitigating factor is the extent to which the patient can avoid a too close contact with a highly emotional relative. The most clear-cut measure of this is the number of hours per week that the patient spends in actual face-to-face contact with the relatives. In our previous study we found that thirty-five hours per week was the critical period; above this, the chances of relapse were greatly increased. The same held true in the present analysis. Several other findings contributed towards a strong impression that social withdrawal could be a protective factor, particularly for unmarried patients.

9 Behavioural observations on parents anticipating the death of a child

Stanford B. Friedman, Paul Chodoff, John W. Mason, & David A. Hamburg*

[*This version of this paper is a heavily abstracted one with considerable detail being cut from most of the early sections. The parents described in the study are broadly representative of major racial, socio-economic status, and religious groups in the USA. A final section on 'Implications for clinical practice' has been deleted. The authors are senior research psychiatrists and pediatricians in the USA.*]

The present paper is concerned with clinical impressions of the response of parents to the impending death of one of their children, gained over a two-year study of the adrenal-cortical response under conditions of chronic psychological stress.

The forty-six subjects represented one or both parents of twenty-seven children all of whom had been referred for treatment with chemo-therapeutic agents to the Medicine Branch of the National Cancer Institute.

Thirty-five parents, twenty mothers and fifteen fathers, lived some distance from the National Institute of Health and were admitted to a ward of the National Institute of Mental Health, where they resided during all or a portion of the time their children were hospitalized. Eleven parents, six mothers and five fathers, who lived in the immediate vicinity of the NIH were available for study to a lesser extent and were seen on what we have considered an 'out-patient' basis.

* extracted from *Pediatrics* (1963) **32** (4) part 1: 610–25

The period of observation for the parents living on the ward ranged from approximately one week to eight months; two months was the median time for the mothers and one month for the fathers. The parents spending a total of four to eight months on this ward had their stay interspersed with periods at home when their children were ambulatory.

The parents studied in the ward setting were interviewed by one of the investigators (S.B.F.) in his office at least once a week and were seen on the ward almost daily. In addition to these interviews and observational notes, the nurses on the 'normal volunteer' ward made and recorded observations, and each morning the parents filled out a brief questionnaire regarding their activities during the previous twenty-four hours.

The interviews were primarily concerned with each parent's perception of his child's illness and clinical course, the defences utilized by the parent to protect him from the impact of the stressful situation and the threatened loss, and the individual's ways of dealing with the many problems that arise when caring for a seriously ill child.

Early reactions of parents

Learning the diagnosis

In general, the parents stated that they had some prior knowledge about leukemia and therefore suspected their child might have this disease before actually hearing it from a doctor and, in this sense, they somewhat anticipated the news. However, without exception, the parents recalled a feeling of 'shock' or of being 'stunned' when hearing the definitive diagnosis. Only an occasional parent reported a concomitant feeling of disbelief, though in retrospect most parents feel that it took some days before the meaning of the diagnosis 'sank in'. Thus, in this study, the majority of parents appeared to intellectually accept the diagnosis and its implication, rather than to manifest the degree of disbelief and marked denial (e.g., Richmond and Weissman 1955) described by others. Only later did they consciously begin to hope that the diagnosis might be in error.

Guilt

Once the diagnosis of leukemia was made, the parents would, almost without exception initially blame themselves for not having paid more attention to the early nonspecific manifestations of the disease. They wondered whether the child would not have had a better chance of responding to therapy if the diagnosis had been made sooner. Although such reactions of guilt were extremely common, and the deep emotional basis of such feelings has been emphasized by others (Richmond and Weissman 1955), most parents in this study readily accepted assurance from the physician that they had not neglected their child.

Seeking information

The ward physician had at least one lengthy interview with the parents shortly after each child was admitted and, later, periodically discussed the child's condition with the parents and was readily available to answer any further questions. The parents were generally aware and appreciative of these efforts, but there remained what appeared to be an insatiable need to know *everything* about the disease. For many weeks there was, characteristically, an extensive search for additional information, especially about therapeutic developments.

This search took many forms, but most noticeable, at least to the medical and nursing staffs, was the exchange of information among parents on the floor solarium which served as a waiting room for the parents between the morning and afternoon visiting hours. Here the 'new' parents would glean information from the group, not only about leukemia and its therapy, but also regarding hospital policies and organization.

The seeking of information can be understood partly as a realistic attempt to learn as much as possible about leukemia in order to better master the situation and care for the ill child. However, the process of learning about leukemia appeared constructive only up to a point, and a sudden upsurge of parental questions often reflected increased anxiety or conflict, which could not be resolved by the acquisition of more detailed information about the disease.

Psychological management of the ill child

The hospitalized child

An almost universal concern of the parents was the question of how much the children knew, or should know, regarding their diagnosis. Anxiety about this problem was considerable, although obviously influenced by the particular parents involved, the age of the child, and the help received in this area from the physician. The majority of parents, even those who realistically accepted the nature of the tragedy, shielded their children from ever hearing the word 'leukemia', though in the hospital setting this was at times all but impossible. Our impression is that *some* acknowledgement of the illness is often helpful, especially in the older child, in preventing the child from feeling isolated, believing that others are not aware of what he is experiencing, or feeling that his disease is 'too awful' to talk about.

The child in remission

Parents would eagerly look forward to the time that their child would go into remission and be discharged from the hospital, but their pleasurable anticipation of this event was frequently tempered by considerable concern regarding the necessity of again assuming the major responsibility for the child's care. They feared that without warning some acute medical problem would arise and any past feelings of inadequacy associated with failure to recognize the original symptoms were re-awakened.

Defense patterns and coping mechanisms

Coping behaviour

Coping behaviour is a term that has been used to denote all of the mechanisms utilized by an individual to meet a significant threat to his psychological stability and to enable him to function effectively.

The 'shock' of learning the diagnosis and the associated lack of emotional experience has already been mentioned, and this may conveniently be classified as an extreme degree of isolation of affect, a mechanism by which the apparent intellectual recognition of a painful event is not associated with a concomitant intolerable emotional response. Only after a few hours or days was there profound emotional feeling and expression associated with the intellectual awareness of what had happened, this usually occurring only after the necessary arrangements had been made for the child's immediate treatment.

Over a period of time the parents became increasingly knowledgeable about leukemia, and would often request rather detailed information regarding their child's condition, especially about laboratory results. Enquiries about a haemoglobin level or leukocyte count were common and, in addition, occasionally such data would spontaneously be given by a doctor in order to help explain the more general situation. This led to attempts, generally unsuccessful, on the part of some parents to predict what therapy their child should receive next, with confusion and suspicion when their 'medical judgement' disagreed with that of the physician. Having once received such detailed information, the parents tended to expect a daily briefing, and would exhibit at first disappointment, then anger, when this routine was interrupted. Such concern over details did serve a defense function by allowing the parents, as well as the doctors, to avoid the more general, but also the more tragic and threatening, aspects of the case. However, our impression was that, over all, more anxiety was generated than dissipated by this practice.

Social influences

The adjustment seen in most of the parents characteristically included a relatively high degree of intellectual acceptance of the diagnosis and prognosis. Realistic arrangements, including those directly related to the care of the ill child, were therefore facilitated. However, this acceptance was not easy to achieve and came about only after a good deal of emotional struggle, expressed as 'We had to convince ourselves of the diagnosis'. It is therefore pertinent that relatives and friends did not usually help in this process, but rather, were more likely to hinder the realization of the child's condition.

Typically, the children's grandparents tended to be less accepting of the diagnosis than the parents, with more distant relatives and friends challenging reality even more frequently. The tendency for the degree of reality-distortion to increase with the remoteness of its source from the immediate family almost made it appear that some of the parents were surrounded by 'concentric circles of disbelief'. Friends and relatives would question the parents as to whether the doctors were *sure* of the diagnosis and prognosis, and might suggest that the parents seek additional medical opinion. Comments would be made that the ill child, especially if he was in remission, could not possibly have leukemia as he looked too well or did not have the 'right symptoms'. Individuals cured of 'leukemia' would be cited and in a few cases, faith healers and pseudomedical practitioners were recommended.

Although parents generally perceived most of these statements and suggestions as attempts to 'cheer us up and give us hope', they found themselves in the uncomfortable position of having to 'defend' their child's diagnosis and prognosis, sometimes experiencing the feeling that others thought they were therefore 'condemning' their own child. Thus, the parents were not allowed to express any feelings of hopelessness. Yet, as will be discussed later, they were paradoxically expected to appear grief-stricken.

Grandparents not only displayed more denial than the parents, but often appeared more vulnerable to the threatened loss of the loved child. Therefore, many of the parents felt that they had to give emotional support to the grandparents at a time when it was most difficult for them to assume this supportive role. Our impression is that this marked degree of emotional involvement on the part of the grandparents helps explain the observations of Bozeman, Orbach, and Sutherland (1955), who noted that the mothers in their study did not often turn to their own mothers for support or guidance. In spite of this, grandparents generally were informed of the diagnosis almost immediately, though parents would occasionally first tell 'people we hardly knew ... just to make sure that we could get through it'.

Though society did not allow the parents to give up the hope that their children might survive, it also assumed that they would be grief-stricken. Therefore, the parents were not expected to take part in normal social activities, or be interested in any form of entertainment. The relatively long course of leukemia made this expectation not only un-realistic, but also undesirable in that some diversion appears necessary in allowing the parents to function effectively in the care of the ill child. Illustrative of this area of conflict was the experience of one mother, whose child had had leukemia for one year. She gave a birthday party for one of her other children and was immediately challenged by relatives who 'could not understand how my family could have a party *at a time like this*'. Such remarks often produced anxiety, guilt, or confusion in a parent, leading this same mother to remark 'that being a parent of a leukemic child is hard, but not as hard as other people make it'.

An additional problem was that friends and relatives often besieged the parents with requests for information about their child. Parents would have to repeatedly describe each new development, listening by the hour to repetitive expressions of encouragement and sympathy, and occasion-ally having to reassure others that the disease was not contagious. This arduous task was ameliorated in the cases where a semi-formal system evolved in which some one individual, often a close friend or a minister, would be kept up to date so that he in turn could answer the multitude of questions.

Although it was clear that friends and relatives sometimes aggravated the parents' distress, they also provided significant emotional support in the form of tactful and sympathetic listening and by offering to be of service, as has been described in detail by Bozeman, Orbach, and Sutherland (1955). The major source of emotional support for most parents during the period of hospitalization appeared to be the other parents of similarly afflicted children, with the feeling that 'we are all in it together' and with concern for the distress experienced by the other parents, a mode of adjustment discussed in detail by Greene and Miller (1958). The parents learned from each other, and could profit by observing the coping behavior manifested by others in the group. Thus, the common fear of 'going to pieces' when their child would become terminally ill was greatly alleviated by watching others successfully, albeit painfully, go through the experience.

Search for meaning

The parents generally found it intolerable to think of their child's leukemia as a 'chance' or meaningless event. Therefore, they tried to construct an explanation for it, displaying a certain amount of urgency until one appropriate to their particular frame of reference could be accepted.

A few parents were content with what might be termed a 'deferred explanation'; that is, they accepted and appeared satisfied with the knowledge that it would be some years before a scientifically accurate answer was available to tell them why *their* child had acquired leukemia. Parents in this category were all relatively well educated and were able to evaluate the current thoughts regarding the etiology of leukemia, coming to the *conclusion* that definitive proof of causation was still lacking. This did not constitute an acceptance of leukemia as a 'chance' phenomenon, but rather implied an ability to wait for the accumulation of more knowledge regarding the etiology of the disease.

A greater number of parents appeared to need a more immediate and definite answer. They would eagerly and unconditionally accept one of the more recent theories concerning the etiology of leukemia, such as the 'viral theory', with some additional explanation as to why it was *this* particular child, rather than some other child, who developed the disease. Most parents constructed an explanation which was a composite of scientific facts, elements from the parents' past experiences, and fantasies. Though in the majority of cases their concept of etiology served to partially resolve any feelings of being responsible for the child's illness, the synthesis sometimes appeared to reflect parental self-blame. In these instances the guilt appeared to be less anxiety-provoking than the total lack of a suitable cause for the leukemia, and therefore guilt may at times be thought of as serving a defense function for the individual.

Hope and anticipatory grief

The element of hope as it refers to a favorable alteration of the expected sequence of events, though hard to evaluate, is of general clinical importance, and was universally emphasized by the parents. Comments would be made such as 'Without hope I could never keep going ... though I know deep down nothing really can be done'. Unlike massive denial, hope did not appear to interfere with effective behavior and was entirely compatible with an intellectual acceptance of reality. That the persistence of hope for a more favorable outcome does not require the need to intellectually deny the child's prognosis is of clinical significance, as it differentiates hope from defense patterns that potentially may greatly distort reality. Hope actually helped the parents accept 'bad news' in that the ward physician would often couple discouraging news with some hopeful comment.

As the disease progressed in the children, there was usually a corresponding curtailment of hope in the parents. Whereas at first they might hope for the development of a curative drug, as the child became increasingly ill, the hope might be only for one further remission. Parents would note that they no longer were making any long-range plans and that they were living on a day-to-day basis. The hopes regarding their children would tend to be so short-term and limited that parents would find themselves preoccupied with a question such as whether their child would be well enough that evening to attend a movie, rather than think about his ultimate fate. This gradual dissipation and narrowing of hope appeared inversely related to the increasing presence of what has been called anticipatory grief.

The process of resigning oneself to the inevitable outcome was frequently accompanied by statements of wishing 'it was all over with'. The narrowing of hope and the completion of much of the grief work was described by one mother who stated: 'I still love my boy, want to take care of him and be with him as much as possible ... but still feel sort of detached from him.' In spite of feeling 'detached' from her child, this mother continued to be most effective in caring for and comforting her child, with no evidence of physical abandonment. Richmond and Weissman (1955) have commented on the usefulness of this anticipatory mourning in step-wise preparing the parent for the eventual loss, and the few parents in our study who did not display such behavior experienced a more prolonged and distressing reaction after the child actually died.

Terminal phase

Terminal episode and death

The parents realized that the clinical condition was much more serious when all of the established chemotherapeutic agents had been exhausted, this event marking what might be considered the beginning of the terminal phase of the illness. Characteristically at this time, there was an acceleration of the grief-work or the actual precipitation of mourning in those few individuals who previously had denied the prognosis, and to the staff, the parents often appeared resigned to the fact that their child would die. Often, as previously described, parents would become increasingly involved in the care of other children on the ward, and occasionally a parent would openly express the desire to resume a more normal life and return to the other children at home. Though these feelings prevailed, there still were residuals of hope, if only that the child might 'just smile once more' or 'have one more good day'. During this terminal period, the knowledge that the doctor 'who knows the case best' would be in daily contact seemed of particular importance. However, in spite of this appreciative attitude, the parents were also less understanding and easily became annoyed when even minor things did not go exactly according to plan. There were apt to be frequent, though brief, expressions of irritation or anger, often followed by spontaneous denial of such feelings. These transient manifestations of hostility might have been related to the direct challenging of an under-lying unrecognized belief in the omnipotent nature of the doctors and the hospital, or in some cases, a displacement of unconscious resentment and ambivalence from the ill child to the medical staff.

In this setting, the child's death was generally taken calmly, but with the appropriate expression of affect. Outbursts of uncontrollable grief or open expressions of self-blame were the exception, and usually there was some indication of relief that the child was no longer suffering. There were arrangements, telephone calls, and decisions to be made, and characteristically the father assumed the more dominant and sup-portive role, just as he had shortly after the diagnosis had first been made.

The death of the child therefore did not appear to be a severe super-imposed stressful situation, but rather an anticipated loss at the end of a long sequence of events. This was also reflected in the seventeen-hydroxycorticosteroid excretion rates, in that there was not one parent who showed a marked rise during the last day of urine collection, which frequently included the time the child had actually died, nor were plasma corticosteroid elevations observed several hours after the child's death. These findings might in part be due to the parents not yet experiencing the emotion, as many of them remarked that they 'just cannot believe that it's all over ... it just hasn't hit yet'.

The parents of the children who died relatively early in our study were invited to return to NIH for a three-day period. Twenty-three parents were thus approached; eighteen, including eight couples, accepted and were seen three to eight months after the end of their children's illness. In addition, three parents who lived in the immediate vicinity of NIH were also available for study during a comparable period.

The grief reactions following the actual loss of the children, as related by these parents, were very similar to, though in some cases not as intense, as those following a sudden loss, and the mourning usually became much less pronounced after three to six weeks. There was a tendency for feelings of guilt and self-blame to be verbalized, often for the first time, and as others have noted, repeated reassurance from the doctor was frequently quite comforting during this period. One might speculate that in some cases an unconscious or barely conscious wish for relief of tension through the child's death during the terminal phase provided the motivation for such expressions of guilt during the mourning period.

Of the eighteen parents who returned to NIH after their child's death, sixteen felt that the return had been a helpful experience. Some of these parents believed that they 'would have been drawn back', even if they had not been invited to again participate in the study. This feeling existed in the face of a 'dread about returning', sometimes accompanied by a tendency to think of their child as still a patient at the hospital. In these parents, there was a feeling of relief soon after arrival at NIH, expressed as 'It wasn't anywhere near as hard as I thought it would be', followed by statements to the effect that returning to NIH 'has put a period on the whole affair ... it now seems more real that Jimmy is not with us'. In our opinion, this suggests that an unconscious remnant of denial persisted in many parents, reflecting a previous denial process that was not always readily apparent when the child was still alive. This apparent acceleration in the termination of the grief process was not reported by two parents who did not appear to have accepted their loss to any significant degree, though approximately six months had elapsed since the death of their children.

Though our follow-up observations are still limited and confined to twenty-one couples, it is known that five mothers became pregnant either during or immediately following their child's illness. There is not sufficient data in three cases to judge whether the pregnancy was planned, but in the other two there was a deliberate effort to conceive. One additional couple attempted to adopt a child approximately four months after their own child had died, and in one other family, the mother is attempting to become pregnant some six months after their youngest child died.

None of the parents who have thus far participated in our follow-up study have reported an increased incidence of somatic complaints or minor illnesses, nor have any of the parents developed any acute medical problems requiring hospitalization subsequent to the actual loss of their child. However, it is recognized that the follow-up period has been of inadequate length to make any statements regarding the possible relationship of unresolvable object loss and the grief reaction to the development of disease, as has been suggested by Schmale (1958) and Engel (1961).

PART IV
Work, life chances, and life styles

10 Social class variations in health care and in the nature of general practice consultations

Ann Cartwright & Maureen O'Brien*

[*This paper has been edited from the original mainly by the deletion of a discussion placing the paper within the framework of an ongoing debate concerning the influence of class on the UK health service. Otherwise editing is according to the editors' general strategy. The authors are research sociologists in the UK.*]

To understand general class variations in the use of health services we need to consider some of the possible mechanisms contributing to differential use.

Mechanisms contributing to differential use of services with social class

There is a problem as to how to take differential needs into account when interpreting differential use of services (Rein 1969a and b). The situation is further complicated because mortality and morbidity rates may indicate *outcomes* of care as well as *needs* for care. Indeed, logically a need for care is dependent on care having some effect – although it need not be in terms of morbidity or mortality, but could be in terms of comfort and the relief of pain and anxiety.

*extracted from M. Stacey (ed.), *The Sociology of the National Health Service* (1976). *Sociological Review* Monograph No. 22. Keele: University of Keele

A review of inequality and the health service was presented recently by Townsend (1974). He discussed the twin themes of inequality in health conditions or needs (looking at infant mortality, life expectation, measurements of physique, and self reported morbidity) and of provision of services. One mechanism he identified was the unequal distribution of resources in relation to population within England.

Unequal geographical distribution of resources

Townsend (1974) commented that 'discussion of inequalities between regions and areas is too often sealed off from discussion of the underlying inequalities of class, income, and housing and living conditions'. Noyce, Snaith, and Trickey (1974) analyzed the expenditure by health authorities in the three branches of the health service 1971–72. They found a significant positive correlation between the percentage of the population in professional and managerial socio-economic groups and both community health expenditure and hospital expenditure. There was a negative correlation between the percentage of the population in un-skilled and semi-skilled manual socio-economic groups and both community health and hospital revenue expenditure. They conclude 'evidently as late as 1971–72 no effort was achieving success in directing new capital to deprived regions'. And 'where these (social class V) people are most abundant fewest resources are available'. The study of Noyce, Snaith, and Trickey was based on regional variations. A more recent one by Buxton and Klein (1975) showed that variations between Area Health Authorities are far more important than those between regions. Hart (1971) also discussed the uneven distribution of care and its historical background. He summed his findings up in the 'inverse care law – the availability of good medical care tends to vary inversely with the need for it in the population served'. Some of the mechanisms he identified were:

(1) 'The origins of the general practitioner service in industrial and coal mining areas.'
(2) The over representation of professional families among medical students.
(3) Doctors 'most able to choose where they will work go to middle-class areas and ... the areas with highest mortality and morbidity tend to get those doctors who are least able to choose where they will work'. This is partly because 'the better-endowed, better-equipped, better-staffed areas of the service draw to themselves more and better staff, and more

and better equipment and their superiority is compounded'.

(4) 'The career structure and traditions of our medical schools [which] make it clear that time spent at the periphery in the hospital service, or at the bottom of the heap in industrial general practice, is almost certain disqualification for any further advancement.'

More recently Hart (1972), commenting on occupational mortality data, draws attention to the fact that mortality differences by social class are increasing.

Knowledge and education

Knowledge of the nature of illness should enable people to use health services more effectively and appropriately. And what data there are suggest that the middle class are more knowledgeable than the working class.

(1) The proportion of people giving four or five right answers to questions about whether diabetes, anaemia, bronchitis, tuberculosis, and polio were catching fell from 82 per cent of people in social class I to 53 per cent in social class V (Dunnell and Cartwright 1972).

(2) Middle-class children were more likely to learn the facts of life earlier than working-class children (Schofield 1965).

(3) The proportion of mothers who thought withdrawal the most reliable method of birth control rose from 1 per cent of those with professional husbands to 10 per cent of those with husbands in skilled jobs. There was also a clear trend in the proportion who thought the pill most reliable, from 79 per cent in the professional class to 50 per cent in the unskilled. in addition, the proportion of mothers who felt they knew as much as they would like to about different methods of contraception fell from 63 per cent of those with husbands in professional jobs to 35 per cent of those with husbands doing unskilled work, and the proportion who had not heard of the IUD, coil or loop rose from 8 per cent to 37 per cent (Cartwright 1970).

(4) The proportion of people who disagreed that a daily bowel movement was important for keeping healthy fell from 37 per cent in social class I to 7 per cent in social class V (Dunnell and Cartwright 1972).

There are, in addition, several American studies that are not quoted here – but with findings in the same direction.

An illustration of the way education may relate to the use of health services is provided by Cameron and Hinton (1968). For patients admitted to hospital for operations on the breast they found a tendency for earlier consultation among patients who had stayed on at school longer.

Attitudes, self-confidence, and diffidence

There is a certain amount of evidence to show that middle-class patients are more critical of services although they are probably better served:

(1) Professional people were the most critical and unskilled people the least critical about their doctor having a well-equipped, up-to-date surgery, having a pleasant, comfortable waiting room, and explaining things to them fully (Cartwright 1967).

(2) Middle-class hospital patients said they were not able to find out all they wanted to know more often than did the working-class ones, and within the working class the skilled people said this more frequently than the semi-skilled, and the semi-skilled more than the unskilled. However, when all those expressing some dissatisfaction are combined, these differences between the social classes disappear (Cartwright 1964).

The conclusion from this last observation was that 'working-class patients may be more diffident about expressing criticism, and also possibly less articulate about their difficulties in communication'.

There are quite a lot of data suggesting that middle- and working-class patients have similar hopes and reactions to their doctors but that the working-class patients are more diffident about asking for information.

One study found that the descriptions of the personal characteristics of their doctor that they appreciated – his willingness to listen, to explain things, to give them confidence, his approachability, his straightforwardness – did not vary to any great extent with social class (Cartwright 1967). Another survey of hospital patients found no difference between the middle- and working-class patients in the proportion who said that when they were ill they liked to know as much as possible about their illness, but the proportion who said they liked to know the details, as well as how it affected them, rose from 24 per cent of the unskilled people to 54 per cent of the professional (Cartwright 1964). This same study also illustrated the greater diffidence of the working class; 'Patients in the professional class were more likely to ask questions, while those in the unskilled manual group more often waited to be told'.

Vulnerability

A recent study by Brown, Harris and Ní Bhrolcháin (1975) was concerned with social class differences in events with severe long term threatening implications which they had previously shown (Brown, Harris, and Peto, 1973) play an important role in bringing about depressive and other affective disorders in women. They found that more working-class than middle-class women had experienced a recent 'severe life-event' but this only explained a small part of the social class differences in the prevalence of depressive symptoms. A larger part of the difference seemed to be explained by a greater likelihood of working-class women breaking down once one of the 'life events' had occurred.

They identified four factors which increase the chances of developing a psychiatric disorder when an event occurs: loss of mother in childhood, three or more children aged under fourteen living at home, lack of an intimate confiding relationship with a husband or boyfriend, and lack of full- or part-time employment. They found 'the first three were more common in the working class and between them they explain the class difference in vulnerability'.

The nature of general practitioner consultations

Up to now the mechanisms we have been considering operate mainly in the community or the hospital. In the last part of this paper we look at some data about the nature of general practitioner consultations and the way this varies in relation to social class.

If working-class patients are more hesitant than middle-class people about asking questions and have more difficulty about expressing their problems in ways they feel will be acceptable to their middle-class doctors then it may take longer, in terms of the length of the consultation or the number of consultations for working-class patients and general practitioners to communicate efficiently. A higher consultation rate may simply be a reflection of this difficulty. To examine this hypothesis consultations need to be studied in depth. Two recent studies have attempted this. Buchan and Richardson (1973) observed and timed 2,113 consultations classifying the various activities of the doctor. Cartwright, Lucas, and O'Brien (1974) tape-recorded ninety-two consultations with elderly patients, interviewed the patients three times – before they saw the doctor, immediately afterwards, and ten days later in their own homes – and also interviewed the doctor at the end of the surgery session. The data presented here on social class variations in this last study have not previously been published.[1]

The consultations

Buchan and Richardson found a clear social class gradient in the 'face-to-face' duration of the consultation from an average of 6.1 minutes for those in social class I (professionals) to 4.4 minutes for those in social class V (the unskilled workers).

In our study, too, the average length of conversation time[2] was greater at consultations with middle-class patients than with working-class ones, 6.2 minutes on average compared with 4.7 minutes. But we found no differences in the proportions who received repeat or other prescriptions, or in those who were examined.

More problems were discussed at consultations with middle-class patients than at those with working-class patients: an average of 4.1, compared to 2.8. And, although working-class patients were rather more likely to say they would ask their doctor's advice about a personal problem the proportion of problems which were social rather than medical was similar for the two groups – 13 per cent.

While the middle-class patients discussed more problems at the consultation, when we asked about a list of complaints which are fairly common among elderly people it certainly did not appear that this was because the middle class perceived themselves as having more problems. If anything, the difference was the other way round although it might have occurred by chance. Middle-class patients reported an average of 2.2 symptoms against 3.0 for working-class. This suggests that middle-class patients were more inclined to discuss their problems with the doctor. Analysis of the communications during the consultation suggests some of the ways in which this might happen.

Communications at consultations

In our study middle-class patients did not talk for a larger proportion of the consultation time, but there was some indication that they asked slightly more questions, an average of 3.7, compared with 3.0, and gave more pieces of information (thirty-six pieces compared with thirty for working-class patients), but neither of these differences reached a level of statistical significance.

Sometimes doctors cut short discussion of further problems, and the following examples illustrate some of the ways in which they did this.

Doctor: Apart from these palpitations you're really very healthy, aren't you?
Patient: Yes, yes. Well, I mean, I have varicose veins you know.
Doctor: Oh yes.
Patient: And I've got a small ulcer, but it's dry now.
Doctor: Mm.
Patient: On my right leg I have a small ulcer.
Doctor: Yes, that's very good.
Patient: But it's drying up gradually. One day I think it's gone completely but it hasn't. It comes back. But...
Doctor: Now here's the letter to see about your eyes.

An example of the ways doctors encouraged people to bring up additional problems or symptoms comes from the early part of a consultation:

Doctor: You've been spitting blood?
Patient: Yes.
Doctor: It comes when you cough?
Patient: Yes but not always.
Doctor: Any other trouble?
Patient: Well, when I've taken that medicine I've been prescribed that all comes up with it.
Doctor: Have you noticed any other trouble at all?
Patient: In what way?
Doctor: Any other complaints?
Patient: No.
Doctor: Any pains anywhere?
Patient: No.
Doctor: Any trouble with your joints or your hands?'
Patient: Only my feet.

One possible indication that doctors may be more inclined to cut short working-class patients more frequently than middle-class ones is that they felt working-class patients more often asked them about inappropriate problems. The doctors felt they were the most appropriate person to help with all the problems discussed at 93 per cent of the consultations with middle-class patients, but only 83 per cent of the ones with working-class patients. (A difference that might well occur by chance – more than once in ten times.)

The doctor–patient relationship

The single consultations we studied related to one point in time in a continuing relationship and can therefore only give a limited picture of the relationship. But the data indicate that some aspects of this relationship differed between working-class and middle-class patients. Working-class patients tended to have been with the practice for longer, an average of 13.9 years compared to 10.1 years for middle-class patients. This might suggest that working-class patients would know their doctors better than middle-class patients, and that the doctors would also be more familiar with their working-class patients. In fact this did not appear to be so; 80 per cent of middle-class patients felt the doctor would know them by name if he met them on the street compared to 72 per cent of working-class patients, and the doctors themselves said they would know 90 per cent of middle-class patients and 81 per cent of working-class patients if they met them on the street – statistically insignificant differences but in the opposite direction to what might be expected from their length of time in the practice. There was no difference in the number of times the two groups had consulted the doctor during the previous twelve months.

There were also variations in how much the doctors knew about the domestic situations of their patients. They did not know whom 15 per cent of their working-class patients lived with; this figure was only 4 per cent for middle-class patients.

Conclusions

The studies we have considered cover a wide range of health services but are by no means comprehensive. Much of the data come from enquiries in which social class differences were not a central theme. There appears to us to be fairly conclusive evidence that the middle class make more use of preventive services. There is also enough evidence to suggest that the middle class may, in relation to a number of services, receive better care. One of the reasons for this is the uneven distribution of services. Another appears to be the greater ability of the middle class to communicate with doctors effectively.

As doctors are themselves middle class, one might expect them to communicate more easily with their middle-class patients, and much of the data support this. General practitioners knew more about the domestic situation of their middle-class patients, although working-class patients had been with them for longer. Middle-class patients discussed more problems and spent longer in conversation with the doctor. The may also ask more questions and give more information.

On these criteria middle-class patients appear to have a more satisfactory relationship with their doctors, but at the same time they are more critical of the care they are given. These two observations do not seen inconsistent. As Titmuss (1968) put it ten years ago 'higher standards of education in the nation as a whole and a more sophisticated adult population are likely to herald the gradual disappearance of an uncomplaining, subservient, class-saturated acceptance of low standards of professional service'.

Notes

1 There are some difficulties in classifying elderly people in terms of social class. A replication on a different sample is therefore desirable.
2 We took the total length of the consultation and subtracted the time when neither patient nor doctor was talking, for instance when examinations were being carried out, and also any time the doctor spent in extraneous conversation, e.g., talking on the telephone or to his receptionist. This gave us the conversation time.

11 Clash in perspective between worker and client

John E. Mayer and Noel Timms*

[*This paper has been reduced from the original by only a small amount in accordance with the editors' general strategy. The authors are a sociologist working in the US and Professor of Social Work in the UK, respectively.*]

For many years caseworkers have experimented with different ways of helping people. Curiously, the resultant innovations have stemmed not from the client's perception of what is helpful, but from the practitioner's. Moreover, with few exceptions the effectiveness of help has been judged by the persons offering, not receiving help. In a word, the client has rarely been asked what kind of help he wants or what he thinks of the help he has been given.

In 1967 the client's point of view was explored in interviews with sixty-one persons who had recently been clients of a voluntary social work agency, the Family Welfare Association of London, formerly the Charity Organization Society (Mayer and Timms, 1970). All the respondents had been born in the British Isles and were living in London at the time. With few exceptions, they had a working–class background. The research interview was semi-structured and centred primarily on the following areas: the events leading the client to the agency; the client's

* extracted from *Social Casework* (1969): 32–40, January

impressions of the social workers and of casework; and especially the conditions that led the client to feel satisfied or dissatisfied. The research interview generally lasted about an hour and a half; it was conducted in the client's home and was tape-recorded. The aim was to learn something about the kinds of factors affecting clients' impressions of, and reactions to, casework treatment. The degree to which such factors are typical or atypical of clients in general, whether in England or in the United States, is a separate question that cannot be answered by exploratory studies of this nature.

Only clients who sought help in dealing with another person and were dissatisfied are discussed in this article. While the number of such cases is small (15/61), the conclusions reached are frequently supported by the material gathered from other clients.

The clients' expectations

Prior to coming to the agency, the clients envisioned the worker as some-one who would be unbiased, educated, and experienced in dealing with personal problems. They expected the worker to listen to their story and after one or possibly two sessions reach a conclusion based on right and wrong. Mrs A., for example, who felt wronged by her husband, did not know whether it was proper for her to leave him because of her obligations to her children. She fully expected the worker to point out the right course to follow. Other wives, including wives who had no thought of leaving their husbands, expected the worker, after learning of their marital troubles, to arrive at a moral assessment. Referring to her description of how she had treated her husband, Mrs L. remarked, 'I thought they'd tell me whether I was doing right or wrong'.

The clients' anticipation of such judgements does not necessarily imply that *they* had any doubt about who was right and who was wrong. Typically, they thought they were right, and they fully expected the worker to agree with them. Nevertheless, they conscientiously tried to describe their situations dispassionately. Presumably they did so because they believed it was the correct way to act in the presence of a judge – the outside authority who renders an impartial decision. Furthermore, they may have thought that it was in their interest to present themselves as reasonable, just, tolerant persons so that their allegations would appear more credible.

It is significant that the clients did not usually expect the worker's activity to end simply with the making of a moral assessment. On the contrary, they fully expected the worker also to assist in rectifying the situation by helping them to implement his decisions. The clients took it for granted that the only way to improve the situation was to bring about changes in the offender's behaviour. They anticipated help from the social worker in either of two ways. He could instruct the client in ways of acting that would lead the culprit to behave differently. Expectations of this nature were clearly held by Mrs F., who stated:

> 'I can easily tell you what I thought it would be like going to the agency. I would bare my soul and my reactions to what my husband did and said. I would hold nothing back, like I do with the neighbours. I would tell the lady all the nasty things that I did back to Brian, and I thought she would say, "If you didn't say this or react like that, Brian wouldn't react like he does". As for Brian, I was hoping that they would tell him, "Well, if you didn't treat Mary like that, she wouldn't lose her temper and scream and go into hysterics". It would have helped build something out of the marriage if the woman had said, "You shouldn't have said that" or "You shouldn't have done that" or "I think your marriage would work if you didn't do that, Mary, or if you didn't do that, Brian".'

Most clients hoped that the worker would do more than instruct, that he would deal directly with the offender. For example, the worker could try to draw the husband into treatment and make him 'see the way things are' and, if necessary, 'drum some sense into his head'.

These working-class clients apparently spent little time trying to ferret out the causes of their problems, unlike persons of middle-class background who see many causal possibilities and who believe it is essential to identify the correct ones. To these particular clients, the cause of the trouble was obvious – it was the other person. Before coming to the agency, they typically had dealt with personal problems by bringing pressure to bear on the other person whenever possible. The fact that they had sought professional help in no sense implied a loss of faith in their techniques. Rather, they had sought professional help because they hoped the caseworker would prove to be more effective in wielding techniques that were essentially the same.

The clients' reactions

The clients reacted, at least initially, to the workers' insight-oriented approaches with surprise and puzzlement. They were bewildered by certain aspects of the workers' behaviour and frequently commented on the lack of active participation. The following comment typifies the clients' attitude:

'The welfare lady came to the house one day when my husband was home and there was a big row between us. I got up to it with my husband and he got up to it with me. The welfare lady knew very well what I went through with my husband, but she just sat there and listened, and she never tried to do anything. She just listened and didn't drum any sense into my husband at all.'

The non-activist approach of the workers and their emphasis on talk was not the only thing that surprised and puzzled the clients. Frequently they were taken aback by the worker's tendency to focus on them rather than the person they thought was responsible for the difficulty. Mr and Mrs S., for example, had been very concerned because their sixteen-year-old daughter often quit jobs and stayed out late at night and did not tell her parents where she was. The parents finally turned to the agency in the hope that someone would get through to Penny and make her realize how silly she had been. It is evident from Mrs S.'s report of her experiences that the worker viewed the problem as related more to the parents than to the daughter. 'The social worker wanted to know all about our background when we were young and all that, and I said to my husband, "Well, to my opinion, that's nothing to do with it."'

After their fourth interview Mr and Mrs S. dropped out. Mrs S. gave the following explanation:

'When we came out of there the fourth time, my husband said, "What do you think of it?" and I said, "I don't know what to think of it". Then my husband said, "He just don't give you any idea what he's going to do or anything. Penny's the problem, not us".'

The tendency of practitioners to probe into the past was seen as still another puzzling aspect of their approach. Mrs C. thought such activities had little to do with solving her problems. When the social worker delved into her background, Mrs C. replied:

'Well, she was trying to be helpful, but she wasn't. She was more like a person that was going into you mentally. I can't explain it. She kept asking me about my background and all that – about things that were bothering me when I was a young girl. But that's got nothing to do with what's going on now. Well, that wasn't going to solve my problems, was it? I mean, it's *now*. I'm grown up now.'

The clients' explanations

Understandably the clients tried to make sense of the treatment situation. They tried to find reasons for the strange and totally unfamiliar actions of the social workers. Several different reasons were offered in explanations of their behaviour.

Some clients reasoned that their workers were simply not interested in them and therefore not overly anxious to help them. Mrs A. came to this conclusion, remarking:

> 'Once I got talking to the social worker, I felt at ease, but then I realized that she wasn't entering into what I was saying at all. And I thought, You are not really listening to me. You are not really interested. She just wasn't giving me an answer or any advice at all ... She just kept saying, "Yes, yes" in a quiet sort of way and nodding her head and would I like to come back and that sort of thing.'

Other clients concluded that the workers did not understand their difficulties and therefore failed to deal with the problems effectively and realistically.

It should be added that the caseworkers were not necessarily blamed for their inability to understand. The clients assumed that only persons who had had similar experiences could possibly comprehend what it was like. And, on the basis of this assumption, they typically preferred workers of the same age, marital status, and sex as themselves.

Several clients assumed that the workers distrusted the authenticity of their stories and for this reason failed to take any action. One such client, Mrs B., told the interviewer:

> 'I was disappointed when the social worker remarked, "We don't give advice, as you notice. Also I don't really know you." Which of course she did not, to be fair – as it was the first time I had come in. But with the training that I understand these welfare officers have, they must be a pretty good judge of character ... The point is, I personally can judge whether I would trust a person or not ... If you came to me with problems I would listen to your problems. And if I felt it was genuine and quite honest, I would give an advice there and then as to what should be done.'

Several clients were of the opinion that, because of the conflicting stories of the client and the spouse, the workers did not know how to proceed and therefore did nothing. Mrs C. stated, 'The social worker listened to my husband's side and to mine, but she just didn't come to a decision about what to do. She just couldn't tell who was right and who was wrong.'

Finally, in the opinion of some clients, lack of authority prevented the worker from acting in a 'reasonable' manner. The clients recognized, in varying degrees, that the authority of a social worker was limited. They knew, for example, that a social worker could not insist that a husband come to the agency or force a husband to relinquish his wages to his wife. Significantly, these clients tended to believe that the worker would employ such measures if given the opportunity because, in their judgement, the worker was actually in agreement with them.

The reasons clients gave for the workers' failure to act in a so-called appropriate manner are of interest. They strongly suggest that the clients were almost totally unaware that the workers' approach to problem-solving was fundamentally different from their own. The clients tacitly assumed that the workers shared their approach. They therefore proceeded to find special reasons why the workers' actions had not been guided by it. In other words, the clients attributed their own cultural perspective to their caseworkers, in much the same way that persons of middle-class background occasionally attribute their perspective to working-class persons.

It can be speculated that these explanations played an important part in influencing the clients to drop out. The clients who felt that the worker was not interested in them or did not trust them became angry and resentful – and in developing such feelings moved closer to terminating contact. The clients who concluded that the worker did not understand, was confused, or lacked authority seemed to resign themselves to the fact that the workers would be unable to help. There was little point, therefore, in continuing treatment.

The study implications

The findings of this study are congruent with and yet go beyond those of previous studies concerned with the reactions of working-class persons to psychotherapy. It has been stated that members of the working class do not understand psychotherapeutic processes; that they attribute personal difficulties to external conditions; that they expect the therapist to give advice and take an active role; and that they lack the conceptual and linguistic skills to maintain themselves in a psychotherapeutic encounter (Hollingshead and Redlich 1958; Brill and Storrow 1964; McMahon 1964; Overall and Aronson 1964). Many of these findings were also brought out in our data. However, our interviews with the clients enabled us to see, or at least suggest, that the so-called in-adequacies in the problem-solving thinking of working-class persons are actually by-products or derivatives of a *different system*. In other words, the behaviour of those clients, when viewed in its proper context and not by middle-class standards, becomes more understandable and in many ways very reasonable. Benjamin Paul's remarks in regard to what happens when one cultural system is used as a basis for describing another are pertinent. He states, 'One system ... seems to dissolve or fragment the second system, so that the other group's ways of behaving and thinking appear as an illogical patchwork' (Paul and Miller 1955: 471).

It is our impression that the social workers were unaware that the clients entered the treatment situation with a different mode of problem-solving and that the clients' behaviour during treatment was in part traceable to this fact. In the research interviews with the workers, the clients' behaviour was interpreted by the workers largely, and some-times nearly exclusively, in psychodynamic terms. The workers con-sistently viewed discontinuance as stemming from anxieties aroused by treatment; in other words, the clients could not look at the ways in which they were contributing to the problem. Viewed from a distance, the worker–client interactions have the aura of a Kafka scene: two persons ostensibly playing the same game but actually adhering to rules that are private.

PART V
Becoming a patient

12 The mobile health clinic: a report on the first year's work

*Joseph D. Epsom**

[*This paper has been reduced from the original by only a small amount in accordance with the editors' general strategy. The author, now a Consultant Medical Adviser, was the Medical Officer for the London Borough of Southwark, UK, from 1965 to 1974. The author wishes to acknowledge the help and support of the London Borough of Southwark and its Health Committee, chaired in 1969 by Councillor Mrs L. M. Clum.*]

In 1965 in Southwark 'well-women' clinics were commenced. At these clinics a full gynaecological examination is carried out for women between the ages of twenty-five and sixty; urine testing, blood pressure readings and breast examinations are also carried out and cervical smears are taken. So far each year approximately one-third of the women seen at 'well-women' clinics were found to have some pathology.

In 1967 it was decided to open advisory and preventive clinics for Southwark's over-sixties age group, and since January 1968, three sessions each week have been held in various clinics in the Borough. These clinics have proved successful with the 'senior citizens'.

In mid-1969 the population of Southwark was approximately 295,000; it was estimated there were 65,000 children aged sixteen and under, and 50,000 people aged sixty and over. This means that there were approximately 180,000 people between the ages of sixteen and sixty,

*extracted from a mimeo published by the London Borough of Southwark Health Department 1969

or 60 per cent of the population, who did not have the opportunity of a routine health check.

As a logical extension of the introduction of 'well-women' clinics, and advisory clinics for the over-sixties, the Council decided to carry out a pilot health survey of the general public of the Borough aged between sixteen and sixty. However, before this decision was taken, much preparatory work was necessary. In 1965, following the formation of the new London Borough of Southwark, it was decided to set up advisory committees to assist in the formulation of health policies for this complex area, which comprised three former Metropolitan Boroughs and parts of two former London County Council Health Divisions and some dozen hospitals, including Guy's, the Maudsley, and a large part of the catchment area of King's College Hospital. The Advisory Committees were composed of representatives of the local general practitioners and hospital consultants – the committees covered such fields as psychiatry, geriatrics, gynaecology, etc. In addition, advice was given by Professor Anderson of King's College Hospital, and Professor Butterfield of Guy's Hospital. Informal talks were also held with the then Ministry of Health.

It was decided that the best method of carrying out the survey was by means of a mobile clinic, and approval for this project was given under the Health Visitor and Social Work (Training) Act, 1962.

The survey

The survey consists, for persons aged sixteen to sixty years, of:

(1) A social history, normally taken by the health visitor before the patient's visit to the clinic, and a medical history, normally taken by the clinic nurse immediately prior to the medical examination. These histories are taken on special forms which were designed after full consultation with the Advisory Committee mentioned previously.

(2) A series of tests: haemoglobin estimation (under 80 per cent was considered as a disability); blood pressure; urine testing (labstix); vision (acuity 6/12 or less with or without glasses was considered as a disability); measurement of height and weight (more than 10 per cent above or below ideal weight for sex, age, and height, according to standard tables was considered as a disability); for women over twenty-five there was a full gynaecological examination and a cervical smear.

Arrangements have been made for all blood specimens and

abnormal urine specimens to be tested at local hospitals; there is full cooperation with the hospitals in this matter.

(3) A comprehensive general medical examination by the clinic doctor.

(4) X-ray of chest – attenders are referred to the frequent regular sessions of the South-East London Mass X-ray Service.

The purpose of these tests is to help identify those people who have health and social problems amenable to some form of treatment. It must be emphasized that no treatment is given at the clinic, but the results of all tests are notified to the general practitioner concerned. Patients are advised, where necessary, to visit their family doctor for the results of the examination.

The mobile health clinic

The mobile health clinic is a specially fitted twenty-two foot production-line caravan built to health department specifications at a cost of only £998. The caravan is fully equipped and comprises a reception/waiting room; a nurse's working area which includes a sink unit and wash-hand basin with water heater and two changing/toilet cubicles for use by attenders; and a medical examination room for the doctor, which includes a wash-hand basin, examination couch, desk, and storage facilities. Heating and hot water are provided by means of a calor gas system.

The clinic is staffed by a medical officer (local general practitioners undertake some sessions), a clinic nurse, and a clinic auxiliary. General administrative services are provided at the health department's main offices.

The mobile health clinic visits each of the fifteen (infant welfare clinic) areas of the Borough in turn, and sites immediately convenient to the dwellings of those groups taking part are arranged approximately four weeks in advance. The clinic is based at each site usually for one week, during which ten sessions are held.

The procedure

An efficient procedure is essential in a scheme of this nature, and in order to achieve this aim and to reduce inconvenience to the attender to a minimum, an appointments system is in operation. Ten appointments are made for each session and male and female attenders are seen on separate days. It is very important that the appointment system is adhered to, because the main success of the project is that the clinic doctor has time in which to carry out a full medical examination. Following the distribution of leaflets to homes in the designated areas, the health visitor visits each home, gives further information if required, and books appointments on the spot. Appointments can be made also by ringing the health department head office, in which case the person is put in contact with the health visitor who is responsible for the appointments list.

In view of the age group under survey, i.e., those of employable age, and the need to utilize fully the clinic by whole-time day operation, it was anticipated that the majority of those coming forward would be women. Consequently, four days in each week were reserved for female attenders and one day for male attenders. The sex distribution showed 80 per cent female and 20 per cent male attendances which accurately reflected the anticipated demand from the two groups.

Attendance by social class

It was particularly heartening to find that nearly 35 per cent of the attenders were from social classes IV and V. This compares with 38 per cent for the borough as a whole. There is little doubt that the introduction of a mobile health clinic for the screening survey has contributed to the high proportion of attendances from the lower socio-economic groups. Most other surveys elsewhere showed that persons in groups IV and V were poor attenders.

The results

The survey commenced on November 18, 1968, and by the end of the first year 3,160 persons had attended the mobile health clinic. During this time periodic reviews of administrative and clinical procedures were undertaken and improvements effected where necessary.

It may be seen in *Tables 17, 18*, and *19* that, discounting gynaecological disorders, there were no significant differences in the incidence of illness between males and females, although there were differences in pattern. The incidence for all groups (*Table 18*) showed that only 120 (19 per cent) men and 363 (14 per cent) women out of the total of 3,160 were free from disability; the remaining 2,677 patients had one, or more, disability. Of these 2,677 it was ascertained that 875 (33 per cent) were either receiving treatment for the disability presented or were suffering from a disability of a sufficiently minor nature not to warrant referral to their general practitioner. Nevertheless, 1,802 (57 per cent of the original total) persons were referred to their family doctor for further investigation and possible treatment.

Table 17   *Disability groups*

		16–40 years		41+ years			% age of patients
		M	F	M	F	totals	
cardio-vascular	high blood pressure murmur (for observation (and investigation	33	60	45	199	337	10.6
	by GP hospital) other, e.g., pulse	3	34	5	40	82	2.5
	signs of failure, etc	2	11	5	18	36	1.1
respiratory		10	54	23	62	149	4.7
digestive disorders		83	197	91	199	570	18.0
orthopaedic conditions		17	87	31	247	382	12.0
eye disorders	vision defects	29	142	68	209	448	14.1
	eye diseases	16	18	15	29	78	2.5
teeth and gums		51	145	42	125	363	11.5
nose and throat		21	29	10	18	78	2.5
ear and hearing		13	69	37	113	232	7.3
gynaecological disorders		—	439	—	499	938	29.6
genito-urinary		12	3	3	21	39	1.3
nervous disorders	neurological	8	26	10	27	71	2.2
	psychiatric	14	297	15	190	516	16.3
weight disorders	overweight 10% and above ideal weight	127	416	105	350	998	31.6
	underweight 10% and below ideal weight	24	201	32	157	414	13.1
varicose veins		15	109	42	170	336	10.6
tuberculosis		—	—	—	1	1	0.03
miscel-laneous	hernia	4	7	8	7	26	0.8
	skin	25	97	26	71	219	6.9
	endocrine	1	14	—	17	32	1.0
blood	abnormal hb	—	60	1	63	124	3.9
	abnormal other	—	3	—	1	4	0.1
urinary abnor-malities	protein	3	11	3	4	21	0.7
	glucose	1	1	3	9	14	0.4
	blood	3	22	2	10	37	1.2
	infection	—	5	—	7	12	0.4
cervix uteri carcinoma	suspicious – for observation	—	3	—	3	6	0.2
	in situ (confirmed)	—	3	—	3	6	0.2
	invasive (confirmed)	—	3	—	2	5	0.2
breast	lumps	—	15	—	14	29	0.9
	carcinoma (confirmed)	—	—	—	2	2	0.06
totals		515	2,581	622	2,887	6,605	

Table 18   *Incidence of illness*

| | 16–40 years | | 41+ years | | | % age of patients |
	M	F	M	F	totals	
patients free from disability	77	265	43	98	483	15.3
patients with single disability	126	497	81	223	927	29.3
patients with multiple disability	136	691	165	758	1,750	55.4
totals	339	1,453	289	1,079	3,160	100.0

Table 19   *Sex and age distribution of attenders*

339	1,453	289	1,079	3,160	100.0

Seven cases of pre-invasive cervical cancer, one active case of pulmonary tuberculosis and one confirmed case of carcinoma of the breast are included among the major disorders detected. The types of disability are illustrated in *Table 17*.

Follow-up survey

In order to ascertain what proportion of patients actually received treatment, were placed under observation, or were referred to a hospital or specialist by their general practitioners, it was necessary for follow-up information to be obtained. This was a large and difficult exercise. No less than 115 Southwark general practitioners were involved and it was necessary to cause a minimum of inconvenience to them and to consume as little as possible of their time. In most cases appointments were made for medical officers of the health department to visit the general practitioners' surgeries to obtain the information and, in this connection, the cooperation of the general practitioners was very much appreciated.

For this survey a sample 25 per cent of the total number of patients referred to their general practitioners was followed-up; thus efforts were made to obtain information on 451 of the 1,802 patients referred to their own doctors. The results of this work are given in *Tables 20, 21*, and *22*. *Table 21* illustrates the fact that 37.8 per cent of the survey findings had not previously been known to the GP. *Table 22* demonstrates that 21.8 per cent of the findings made known to the GP for the first time were sufficiently serious to warrant referral to hospital or specialist services.

Table 20   *Attendance results*

	total	%
number of patients who attended GP as requested	405	89.8
number of patients: no confirmation of attending GP; GP retired, ill health, holidays, patient moved away, etc.	46	10.2
total number of patients selected for follow-up survey	451	100.0

Table 21   *Findings*

	total	%
number of Mobile Health Clinic (MHC) findings already known to GP	442	53.4
number of MHC findings not previously known to GP but confirmed by him/her	313	37.8
number of MHC findings not confirmed by GP	73	8.8
total number of MHC findings in respect of the survey patients	828	100.0

Table 22   *Further care arrangements of patients*

	total arrange-ments	%
for observation by GP	147	30.0
for treatment by GP	236	48.2
for referral to hospital or specialist by GP	107	21.8
total number of further care arrangements	490	100.0

Cost per head

The cost per head of the Survey for the First Year's Work (3,160 persons examined as described above) was £2 75p; and compares with private agencies running comprehensive health checks at £25 to £30.

13 Symptom recording and demand for primary medical care in women aged twenty to forty-four years

Michael H. Banks, S. A. A. Beresford,
D. C. Morrell, J. J. Waller,
& C. J. Watkins*

[*The original of this paper contained in addition the analysis and discussion of the influence of anxiety on consultation with doctors. These sections have been removed with the agreement of the authors. The paper is presented together with the previous one primarily to indicate the general background against which theories about 'illness behaviour' must be set. The work was carried out from the Department of Community Medicine of St Thomas's Hospital Medical School, London.*]

Introduction

Many studies have shown that variation in and response to morbidity depend upon susceptibility to disease, demographic characteristics such as age, sex, marital status, education, and occupation, together with a wide range of other personal, social, and cultural factors. The results of this extensive research have been systematically reviewed elsewhere (Kasl and Cobb 1966; McKinlay 1972). It is not intended in this introduction to compete with these reviews, but merely to provide a background to the factors selected for closer scrutiny in this study.

It is predictable that age and sex would affect demand for care in that they affect morbidity, and indeed in the British National Health Service this relationship has been demonstrated in general practice

* extracted from the *International Journal of Epidemiology* (1975) **4** (3): 189–95, where the article appeared under the title, 'Factors influencing the demand for primary medical care in women aged 20–44 years: a preliminary report'.

(Logan and Cushion 1958; HMSO 1974). High consultation rates are characteristic of the very old and the very young, and of women in the age group fifteen to forty-four years. Marital status has been shown to influence the demand for medical care, with widows characteristically requesting care more frequently than married women (Ashford and Pearson 1970). Ashford and Pearson also showed higher utilization of medical care in families of three or more, while Geertsen and Gray (1970) found that mothers of large families were less inclined to assume the sick role than mothers of small families, although favourable attitudes towards a cohesive family network were associated positively with sick-role behaviour.

Educational levels have consistently been demonstrated to influence the demand for medical care. Previous research has shown that lower demands for medical care occur among those who proceeded beyond the age of fifteen in their education (Ashford and Pearson 1970; Rahe, Gunderson, and Ransom 1970; Waller and Morrell 1972). Greater use of preventive services is made by patients with more years of formal education, but emergency services are used less (Kasl and Cobb 1966). Social class affects demand for medical care in complex ways and con-flicting results have been reported (Logan and Cushion 1958; Kedward 1962; Scott and McVie 1962). In the United Kingdom it has been shown that age and social class interact in determining demand for medical care (Dunnell and Cartwright 1972), and in the United States a relationship was demonstrated between social class and the type of medical demand, i.e., preventive versus curative (Kasl and Cobb 1966).

Previous work, using symptom-recall techniques, demonstrated that adults experience symptoms of illness on about one day in four (Dunnell and Cartwright 1972). Only a small proportion of these symptoms lead to a demand for medical care, and it has been shown how demand at the primary care level does not precisely reflect the presence of morbidity (Rea 1972; Morrell 1972; Hull 1969). Differential perception of symptoms and the influence on subsequent illness behaviour has been emphasized previously by Mechanic (1962).

A decision to study women aged twenty to forty-four years was reached as a result of the following considerations:

(a) This age group presents the general practitioner with immediate problems by their unexpectedly high level of demand for medical care, other than demands for obstetric care. That their demands are associated with a high prevalence of psychiatric illness is of particular interest (Morrell, Gage, and Robinson 1970).

(b) This age group is clinically homogeneous in that it does not contain many patients suffering from acute diseases of childhood or chronic degenerative diseases. It seems possible, therefore, that demands for care may be influenced more by behaviour and environment than by disease.

The objectives of this study can be summarized as:

(1) to investigate the relationship between perception of symptoms and demand for medical care.
(2) to determine what factors, independent of perceived symptoms, are associated with demand for care.
(3) to investigate the relationship between these factors and perception of symptoms.
(4) to discover what alternative action to demanding general practitioner care is taken by patients in response to perceived symptoms.

Methodology

Population

A random sample of 516 women aged between twenty and forty-four years was drawn from the general practice age/sex register. Consultations by these women were recorded for a period of twelve months on a special record card inserted in their standard medical records. The data were extracted and coded within forty-eight hours of recording. For the purpose of home interviews each woman was randomly allocated to a month of the year.

Methods of measurement

The following methods of measurement were included in the study:

(i) a social and health questionnaire.
(ii) a forty item anxiety scale.
(iii) a health diary, which the respondent was asked to complete every evening, for four weeks. An example of the lay-out of the diary, which is a modified version of the health calendar used by Roghmann and Haggerty (1972) is given in *Figure 5*. Basically, this diary provides information on perception of symptoms, action taken and the occurrence of special events such as stressful situations.

Figure 5   Health diary

Day	Date Put a ring round the dates of your monthly periods	Has there been anything wrong with you today? If so describe what you noticed wrong.	Did you contact your doctor today? If so, why?	Could you do all your normal activities today?	Did you have to lie down during the day because you felt unwell?	Did you take any medicine today? What was it for and what was its name?	Did you do any-thing else to make yourself feel better? If you did say what.	Did any-thing special happen to you or your family today? If so can you describe what happened?

(iv) general practitioner record card – these cards were inserted in the medical records of the sample population. They provide objective measures of medical care delivered, information on who initiated the consultations, details of presenting symptoms and GP's diagnosis. The use of similar record cards for research purposes has been reported previously by Morrell, Gage, and Robinson (1970), who showed that 47 per cent of all consultations are doctor-initiated. It is clear, therefore, that total consultation rate does not necessarily reflect the patient's decision to seek medical care, and accordingly consultation data has been divided into patient-initiated and doctor-initiated.

Procedure

Each month the women selected were sent a letter inviting them to cooperate in the study. Ten days later they were visited by a field-worker and asked to complete the health diary for a period of four weeks. Two weeks after starting the diary a visit was made to check on the entries and administer the social and health questionnaire. After four weeks, upon completion of the health diary, the Institute of Personality and Ability Testing anxiety questionnaire was administered. Five field-workers were used in all, although not more than two were used at any one time.

The identification data of all 516 women drawn in the sample were checked at the Executive Council, and those who were not currently registered with the practice were withdrawn. Of the 415 remaining women, 19.5 per cent had moved house and attempts by the fieldworkers to discover their new address were unsuccessful, despite the fact that they were still registered with the practice. Before the date allotted to the fieldworker visit 14.9 per cent had left the practice. The doctors excluded 2.2 per cent for reasons of severe marital problems or severe mental illness, leaving 63.4 per cent who were actually contacted. This rate is comparable with other studies in general practice (Hannay 1972; Richardson, Dohrenwend, and Klein 1965).

Results

In the first instance, analysis has been directed towards the simple relationships between perception of symptoms and demand for medical care. For this purpose attention has been restricted to those women who remained registered with the practice for the entire study year and who kept a health diary for at least twenty-one days. There were 198 such women.

As would be expected a certain group of women did not consult with the doctor at all throughout the year. These low utilizers of care amounted to 24 per cent of our sample, and 10 per cent of this group were also symptom-free during the four weeks of their health diary. At the other extreme, two women recorded a symptom on each day of the diary.

A descriptive summary of symptom perception as compared with consultations is presented in *Table 23*.

Table 23   *Symptom episodes and GP consultations*

health diary		consultations with GP	
total days per person	= 28		
mean symptom days per person	= 10	mean annual consultations per person	= 4.71
mean symptom episodes per person	= 6.2		
estimated annual *symptom episodes* per person	= 81	mean annual *patient-initiated consultations* per person	= 2.18

implication: 37 *symptom episodes* to every *patient-initiated consultation*

As can be seen in this table, symptoms were recorded on an average of ten days per diary, which is slightly more frequent than one day in three. An episode of symptoms was defined to be a group of consecutive days on which the same symptom was recorded first. When there was no symptom or a different one recorded, the episode was considered to have terminated. Again, *Table 23* shows that the mean symptom episodes per diary was 6.2; the average length of these episodes was 1.6 days. Making the assumption that there was no bias in the distribution of women keeping their diaries over different months of the year, an extrapolation from the diary experience enabled an estimate of symptom episodes for the entire year to be made. This gave a figure of eighty-one episodes per woman, again shown in *Table 23*.

The consultation records showed a mean number of 4.71 consultations for each woman throughout the year and for patient-initiated consultations the mean number was 2.18. These figures in *Table 23* indicate that for every thirty-seven symptom episodes experienced in this sample of female patients there occurs one patient-initiated consultation.

It is of interest to compare the sort of symptoms experienced by a patient with the symptoms which she presents to the general practitioner. In this study we were able to effect this comparison using the diary record, and the records of the patient-initated consultations. The most frequent symptoms in each case are shown in *Figure 6*. This demonstrates a very marked difference between the distribution of symptoms presented to the general practitioner and those perceived by and acted upon by the patient.

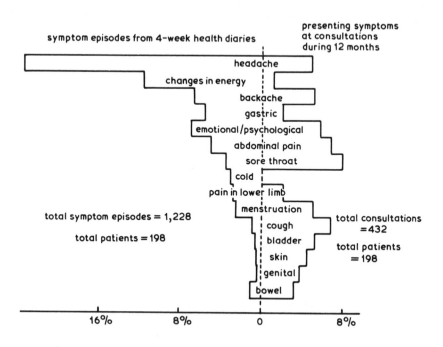

Figure 6   Distribution of common symptoms

Discussion

Ninety-eight per cent of the population of the United Kingdom is registered with National Health Service general practitioners who are obliged by their contract to provide continuing medical care to the patients registered with them. Thus financial considerations do not play a part in the patient's decision to consult, and the majority of self-initiated consultations are made with the patient's own general practitioner.

Several studies have shown that only a small proportion of complaints experienced leads to demands for care. Horder and Horder (1954) and Wadsworth, Butterfield, and Blaney (1971) report that only about a third of illnesses reach a medical agency. Accurate comparisons between the present study and data from previous work are extremely difficult due to differing 'at risk' time periods. However, we know of no other study in Britain that has compared the perception of symptoms as recorded by the patient in a health diary, with symptoms presented by the same patient to the general practitioner. It can be claimed that both these measures are more accurate than those relying on patient recall of symptoms and doctor visits. These results show that only one symptom in thirty-seven led to a consultation, suggesting that the amount of symptomatology managed by patients themselves is greater than previously thought.

Table 24   *Likelihood of symptoms leading to a consultation*

symptoms	number of episodes in 28-day diary period	estimated number of episodes in a year	number of patient-initiated consultations in a year	ratio of symptom episodes to consultations
changes in energy	140	1,825	4	456 : 1
headache	282	3,676	20	184 : 1
disturbance of gastric function	67	873	8	109 : 1
backache	84	1,095	21	52 : 1
pain in lower limb	34	443	9	49 : 1
emotional/psychological	89	1,160	25	46 : 1
abdominal pain	62	808	28	29 : 1
disturbance of menstruation	32	417	21	20 : 1
sore throat	46	600	33	18 : 1
pain in chest	15	196	14	14 : 1

As can be seen from *Figure 6*, the most frequent types of symptoms recorded by the patient and those presented by the patient to the doctor differ markedly. A rank ordering of some of the most common symptoms in terms of their likelihood of leading to a consultation is shown in *Table 24*. It appears that only one episode of headache in 184 leads a patient to consult, but one in eighteen episodes of sore throat leads to a consultation. This suggests an intervening aspect of patient behaviour that evaluates the importance of symptoms in relation to anticipated diagnosis and expectation of treatment. Considering all symptom episodes together the more episodes recorded in the health diary, the more likely the patient is to consult twice or more throughout the year.

14 Pathways to the doctor – from person to patient

Irving Kenneth Zola*

[*This paper has been reduced from the original by only a small amount in accordance with the editors' general strategy. The author is Professor of Sociology in the USA.*]

The problem on which we wish to dwell is one about which we think we know a great deal but that, in reality, we know so little – how and why an individual seeks professional medical aid. The immediate and obvious answer is that a person goes to a doctor when he is sick. Yet, this term 'sick', is much clearer to those who use it, namely the health practitioners and the researchers, than it is to those upon whom we apply it – the patients.

Even when there is agreement as to what constitutes 'sickness' there may be a difference of opinion as to what constitutes appropriate action, as in the following incident:

> A rather elderly woman arrived at the Medical Clinic of the Massachusetts General Hospital three days after an appointment. A somewhat exasperated nurse turned to her and said, 'Mrs Smith, your appointment was three days ago. Why weren't you here then?' To this Mrs Smith responded, 'How could I? Then I was sick.'

Examples such as this are not unusual occurrences. And yet they

*extracted from *Social Science and Medicine* (1973) 7: 677–89 cause little change in some basic working assumptions of the purveyors of medical care as well as the myriad investigators who are studying its delivery. It is to three of these assumptions we now turn: (1) the importance and frequency of episodes of illness in an individual's life; (2) the representativeness of those episodes of illness which come to professional attention; and (3) the process by which an individual decides that a series of bodily discomforts he labels symptoms become worthy of professional attention. Together these assumptions create an interesting if misleading picture of illness. Rarely do we try to understand how or why a patient goes to the doctor, for the decision itself is thought to be an obvious one. We postulate a time when the patient is asymptomatic or unaware that he has symptoms, then suddenly some clear objective symptoms appear, then perhaps he goes through a period of self-treatment and when either this treatment is unsuccessful or the symptoms in some way become too difficult to take, he decides to go to some health practitioner (usually, we hope, a physician).

The first assumption, thus, deals with the idea that individuals at most times during their life are really asymptomatic. The extensive data pouring in from periodic health examination have gradually begun to question this notion. For examinations of even supposedly healthy people, from business executives to union members to college professors, consistently reveal that at the time of their annual check-up, there was scarcely an individual who did not possess some symptom, some clinical entity worthy of treatment (Meigs 1961: 861, Siegel 1963). More general surveys have yielded similar findings (Commission on Chronic Illness 1957; Pearse and Crocker 1954). Such data begin to give us a rather uncomfortable sense in which we may to some degree be sick every day of our lives. If we should even think of such a picture, however, the easiest way to dismiss this notion is that the majority of these everyday conditions are so minor as to be unworthy of medical treatment. This leads to the second assumption; namely, the degree of representativeness, both as to seriousness and frequency, of those episodes which do get to a doctor. Here, too, we are presented with puzzling facts. For if we look at investigations of either serious physical or mental disorder, there seem to be at least one, and in many cases several, people out of treatment for every person in treatment (Commission on Chronic Illness 1957). If, on the other hand, we look at a doctor's practice, we find that the vast bulk is concerned with quite minor disorders. Furthermore, if we use symptom-check-lists or health calendars, we find that for these self-same minor disorders, there is little that distinguishes them medically from those that are ignored, tolerated, or self-medicated.

With these confusions in mind, we can now turn to the third assumption. On the basis that symptoms were perceived to be an infrequent and thus somewhat dramatic event in one's life, the general assumption was that in the face of such symptoms, a rational individual, after an appropriate amount of caution, would seek aid. When he does not or delays overlong, we begin to question his rationality. The innumerable studies of delay in cancer bear witness.

If we examine these studies we find that the reason for delay are a list of faults – the patient has no time, no money, no one to care for children, or take over other duties, is guilty, ashamed, fearful, anxious, embarrassed, or emotionally disturbed, dislikes physicians, nurses, hospitals, or needles, has had bad medical, familiar, or personal experiences, or is of lower education, socio-economic status, or an ethnic or racial minority (Blackwell 1963). As the researchers might put it, there is something about these people or in their backgrounds that has disturbed their rationality, for otherwise, they would 'naturally' seek aid. And yet there is a curious methodological fact about these studies for all these investigations were done on *patients*, people who *had* ultimately decided to go to a physician. What happened? Were they no longer fearful? Did they get free time, more money, outside help? Did they resolve their guilt, shame, anxiety, distrust? No, this does not seem to have been the case. If anything, the investigators seem to allude to the fact that the patients finally could not stand it any longer. Yet given the abundant data on the ability to tolerate pain (Chapman and Jones 1944; Hardy, Wolff, and Goodell 1952) and a wide variety of other conditions, this notion of 'not being able to stand it' simply does not ring true clinically.

We can now restate a more realistic empirical picture of illness episodes. Virtually every day of our lives we are subject to a vast array of bodily discomforts. Only an infinitesimal amount of these get to a physician. Neither the mere presence nor the obviousness of symptoms, neither their medical seriousness nor objective discomfort seems to differentiate those episodes which do and do not get professional treatment. In short, what then does convert a person to a patient? This then became a significant question and the search for an answer began.

At this point we had only the hunch that 'something critical' must ordinarily happen to make an individual seek help. Given the voluminous literature on delay in seeking medical aid for almost every conceivable disorder and treatment, we might well say that the statistical norm for any population is to delay (perhaps infinitely for many). The implementing of this hunch is owed primarily to the intersection of two disciplines – anthropology and psychiatry. The first question to be faced was how and where to study this 'something'. Both prospective and retrospective studies were rejected. The former because as Professor H. M. Murphy noted there is often an enormous discrepancy between the declared intention and the actual act. The retrospective approach was rejected for two reasons – the almost notoriously poor recall that individuals have for past medical experiences and the distortions in recall introduced by the extensive 'memory manipulation' which occurs as a result of the medical interview. Our resolution to this dilemma was a way of studying the patient when he was *in the process* of seeking medical aid. This process was somewhat artificially created by (1) interviewing patients while they waited to see their physician; (2) confining our sample to new patients to the out-patient clinics of the Massachusetts General Hospital who were seeking aid for their particular problem for the first time. Thus, we had a group of people who were definitely committed to seeing a doctor (i.e., waiting) but who had not yet been subject to the biases and distortions that might occur through the medical interview (though some patients had been referred, we included only those on whom no definite diagnosis had been made). This then was where we decided to study our problem.

Given the data on delay in the area of psychiatric illness, it seemed very likely that people have their symptoms for a long period of time before ever seeking medical aid. Thus one could hypothesize that there is an accommodation both physical, personal, and social to the symptoms and it is when this accommodation breaks down that the person seeks, or is forced to seek medical aid. Thus the 'illness' for which one seeks help may only in part be a physical relief from symptoms. The research question on the decision to seek medical aid thus turned from the traditional focus on 'why the delay' to the more general issue of 'why come *now*'. This way of asking this question is in itself not new. Physicians have often done it, but interestingly enough, they have asked it not in regard to general physical illness but rather when they can find nothing wrong. It is *then* that they feel that the patient may want or have been prompted to seek help for other than physical reasons.

The final issue which is essential to understanding the study concerns the nature of the sample. We speculated that ethnic groups, particularly in an area such as Boston, Massachusetts, might well function as cultural reference groups and thus be an urban transmitter and perpetuator of value-orientations, in relation to symptoms. The specific ethnic groups we studied were determined by a demographic survey from which we determined the three most popular ethnic groups at the Massachusetts General Hospital; Italian, Irish Catholic, and Anglo-Saxon Protestant.

To summarize the methodology the sample consisted of patients completely new to the out-patient clinics who were seeking medical aid for the first time for this particular problem, who were between the ages of eighteen and fifty, able to converse in English, of either Anglo-Saxon Protestant, Irish Catholic, or Italian Catholic background. The data collection took place at the three clinics to which these groups were most frequently sent – the eye clinic, the ear, nose, and throat clinic, and the medical clinic, which were, incidentally three of the largest clinics in the hospital. The interviewing took place during the waiting time before they saw their physicians with the general focus of the questioning being: Why did you seek medical aid now? In addition to many such open-ended questions, we had other information derived from the medical record, demographic interviews, attitude scales, and check lists. We also had each examining physician fill out a medical rating sheet on each patient. In all we saw over 200 patients, fairly evenly divided between male and female.

We first examined the presenting complaints of the patients to see if there were differing conceptions of what is symptomatic. Our first finding dealt with the location of their troubles. The Irish tended to place the locus of symptoms in the eyes, the ears, the nose or the throat – sense organs – while the Italians showed no particular clustering. The same result obtained when we asked what was the most important part of the body. Here, too, the Irish tended to place their symptoms in the eyes, ears, nose, and throat with the Italians not favouring any specific location. We noted, however, that this was not merely a reflection of epidemiological differences; for Italians, who did have eye, ear, nose, and throat problems, did not necessarily locate their chief complaint in either the eyes, ears, nose, or throat. We thus began to wonder if this focussing was telling us something other than a specific location. And so we turned our attention to more qualitative aspects of symptoms, such as the presence of pain. Here we noted that the Italians much more often felt that pain constituted a major part of the problem, whereas the Irish felt equally strongly that it did not. However, we had our first clue that 'something else' was going on. The Irish did not merely say they had no pain, but rather utilized a kind of denial with such statements as, 'No, I wouldn't call it a pain, rather a discomfort'; or 'No, a slight headache, but nothing that lasts'. Further analysis of our data then led us to create a typology in which we tried to grasp the essence of a patient's complaint. One type seemed to reflect a rather specific organic dysfunctioning (difficulty in seeing, inappropriate functioning, discharge, or movement, etc) while the second type represented a more global malfunctioning (aches and pains, appearance, energy level, etc). Looked at in this way, we found that significantly more Irish seemed to describe their problem in terms of a rather specific dysfunction whereas the Italians described their complaints in a more diffuse way. Thus, the Irish seemed to convey a concern with something specific, something that has gone wrong or been impaired; whereas the Italians were concerned with or conveyed a more global malfunctioning emphasizing the more diffuse nature of their complaints.

We now had differentiated two ways of communicating about one's bodily complaints – a kind of restricting versus generalizing tendency and we thus sought evidence to either refute or substantiate it. Two 'tests' suggested themselves. The first consisted of three sets of tabulations: (1) the total number of symptoms a patient had; (2) the total number of different types of malfunctions from which he suffered (the typology mentioned above actually consisted of nine codifiable categories); and (3) the total number of different parts of the body in which a patient located complaints. Each we regarded as a measure of generalizing one's complaints. As we predicted the Italians had significantly more complaints of greater variety, and in more places than did the Irish. Our second 'test' consisted of several questions dealing with the effect of their symptoms on their interpersonal behaviour. Here we reasoned that the Irish would be much more likely to restrict the effect of their symptoms to physical functioning. And so it was, with the Italians claiming that the symptoms interfered with their general mode of living and the Irish just as vehemently denying any such interference. Here again, the Irish presented a 'no with a difference' in such statements as 'No, there may have been times that I become uncomfortable physically and afraid to show it socially. If I felt that way I even tried to be a little more sociable.'

The crux of the study is, however, the decision to see a doctor. One of our basic claims was that the decision to seek medical aid was based on a break in the accommodation to the symptoms, that in the vast majority of situations, an individual did not seek aid at his physically sickest point. We do not mean by this that symptoms were unimportant. What we mean is that they function as a sort of constant and that when the decision to seek medical aid was made the physical symptoms alone were not sufficient to prompt this seeking.

In our data we were able to discern several distinct non-physiological patterns of triggers to the decision to seek medical aid. We have called them as follows: (1) the occurrence of an interpersonal crisis; (2) the *perceived* interference with social or personal relations; (3) sanctioning; (4) the *perceived* interference with vocational or physical activity; and (5) a kind of temporalizing of symptomatology. Moreover, these five patterns were clustered in such a way that we could characterize each ethnic group in our sample as favouring particular decision-making patterns in the seeking of medical aid.

The first two patterns, the presence of an interpersonal crisis, and the perceived interference with social or personal relations were more frequent among the Italians. The former, that of a crisis, does not mean that the symptoms have led to a crisis or even vice-versa, but that the crisis called attention to the symptoms, caused the patient to dwell on them and finally to do something about them. An example will illustrate this.

> Carol Conte was a forty-five-year-old, single book-keeper. For a number of years she had been both the sole support and nurse for her mother. Within the past year, her mother died and shortly thereafter her relatives began insisting that she move in with them, quit her job, work in their variety store, and nurse their mother. With Carol's vacation approaching, they have stepped up their efforts to persuade her to at least try this arrangement. Although she has long had a number of minor aches and pains, her chief complaint was a small cyst on her eyelid [diagnosis: fibroma]. She related her fear that it *might* be growing or could lead to something more serious and thus she felt she had better look into it now [the second day of her vacation] 'before it was too late'. 'Too late' for what was revealed only in a somewhat mumbled response to the question of what she expected or would like the doctor to do. From a list of possible outcomes to her examination, she responded, 'Maybe a "hospital"[ization] ... "Rest" would be all right...' [and then in a barely audible tone, in fact turning her head away as if she were speaking to no one at all] 'just so they [the family] would stop bothering me'. Responding to her physical concern, the examining physician acceded to her request for the removal of the fibroma, referred her for surgery, and thus removed her from the situation for the duration of her vacation.

In such cases, it appeared that regardless of the reality and serious-ness of the symptoms, they provide but the rationale for an escape, the calling-card or ticket to a potential source of help – the doctor.

The second pattern – the perceived interference with social or personal relations – is illustrated by another Italian patient.

> John Pell is eighteen and in his senior year of high school. For almost a year he's had headaches over his left eye and pain in and around his right, artificial, eye. The symptoms seem to be most prominent in the early evening. He claimed, however, little

general difficulty or interference until he was asked whether the symptoms affected how he got along. To this he replied, 'That's what worries me ... I like to go out and meet people and now I've been avoiding people'. Since he has had this problem for a year, he was probed as to why it bothered him more at this particular time. 'The last few days of school it bothered me so that I tried to avoid everybody [this incidentally was his characteristic pattern *whenever* his eyes bothered him] ... and I want to go out ... and with my Senior Prom coming up, and I get the pains at 7 or 7.30 how can I stay out ... then I saw the nurse.' To be specific, he was walking down the school corridor and saw the announcement of the upcoming Prom. He noticed the starting time of eight p.m. and went immediately to the school nurse who in turn referred him to the Massachusetts Eye and Ear Infirmary.

In this case, the symptoms were relatively chronic. At the time of the decision there may have been an acute episode, but this was not the first such time the symptoms had reached such a 'state' but, rather, it was the perception of them on this occasion as interfering with the social and interpersonal relations that was the trigger or final straw.

The third pattern, sanctioning, was the overwhelming favourite of the Irish. It is, however, not as well illustrated by dramatic examples, for it consists simply of one individual taking the primary responsibility for the decision to seek aid for someone else. In other words, the Irish seemed to need another person to sanction or give permission to seek help.

There is a secondary pattern of the Irish, which turns out to be also the major pattern of the Anglo-Saxon group. It was almost straight out of the Protestant ethic; namely a perceived interference with work or physical functioning. The word 'perceived' is to be emphasized because the nature of the circumstances range from a single woman, thirty-five-years old, who for the first time noted that the material which she was typing appeared blurred and thus felt that she had better take care of it, to a man with multiple sclerosis who, despite falling down and losing his balance in many places, did nothing about it until he fell at work. Then he perceived that it might have some effect on his work and his ability to continue. The secondary Anglo-Saxon pattern is worth commenting on, for at first glance it appears to be one of the most rational modes of decision-making. It is one that most readers of this paper may well have used, namely the setting of external time criteria. 'If it isn't better in 3 days, or 1 week, or 7 hours, or 6 months, then I'll take care of it.' A variant on this theme involves the setting of a different kind of temporal standard – the recurrence of the phenomenon.

I would now like to note some of the implications of this work. When speaking of implications, I ask your indulgence, for I refer not merely to what leads in a direct line from the data but some of the different thoughts and directions in which it leads me. What for example are the consequences for the very conception of etiology – conceptions based on assumptions about the representativeness of whom and what we study. We have claimed in this paper that the reason people get into medical treatment may well be related to some select social psychological circumstances. If this is true, it makes all the more meaningful our earlier point about many unexplained epidemiological differences, for they may be due more to the differential occurrence of these social-psychological factors, factors of selectivity and attention which get people and their episodes into medical statistics rather than to any true difference in the prevalence and incidence of a particular problem or disorder. Our findings may also have implications for what one studies, particularly to the importance of stress in the etiology of so many complaints and disorders. For it may well be that the stress noted in these people's lives, at least those which they were able to verbalize, is the stress which brought them into the hospital or into seeking treatment (as was one of our main triggers) and not really a factor in the etiology or the exacerbation of the disorder.

Our work also has implications for treatment. So often we hear the terms 'unmotivated, unreachable, and resistance' applied to difficult cases. Yet we fail to realize that these terms may equally apply to us, the caretakers and health professionals who may not understand what the patient is saying or if we do, do not want to hear it. An example of this was seen in the way physicians in this study handled those patients for whose problem no organic basis could be found. For despite the fact that there were no objective differences in the prevalence of emotional problems between our ethnic groups, the Italians were consistently diagnosed as having some psychological difficulty such as tension, headaches, functional problems, personality disorder, etc; whereas the Irish and Anglo-Saxon were consistently given what one might call a neutral diagnosis something that was either a Latinized term for their symptoms or simply the words 'nothing found on tests' or 'nothing wrong'. Our explanation is somewhat as follows, namely that this situation is one of the most difficult for a physician and one in which he nevertheless feels he should make a differential diagnosis. Faced with this dilemma he focussed inordinately on *how* the Italians presented themselves – somewhat voluble, with many more symptoms, and somewhat dramatic social circumstances surrounding their decision to seek help. This labelling of the Italians is particularly interesting since as we mentioned above the Irish and Anglo-Saxons had similar psychological and social problems but presented them in a much more emotionally neutral and bland manner.

One final remark as to treatment; again and again we found that where the physician paid little attention to the specific trigger which forced or which the individual used as an excuse to seek medical aid, there was the greatest likelihood of that patient eventually breaking off treatment. Another way of putting this is that without attention to this phenomenon the physician would have no opportunity to practise his healing art. Moreover, this problem of triggers, etc brooked no speciality nor particular type of disorder. So that being a specialist and only seeing certain kinds of problems did not exempt the physician from having to deal with this issue.

Conclusion

Hopefully, the present research has demonstrated the fruitfulness of an approach which does not take the definition of abnormality for granted. Our data seems sufficiently striking to invite further reason for re-examining the traditional and often rigid conceptions of health and illness, of normality and abnormality, of conformity and deviance. Symptoms or physical aberrations are so widespread that perhaps relatively few, and a biased selection at best, come to the attention of official treatment agencies. We have thus tried to present evidence showing that the very labelling and definition of a bodily state as a symptom as well as the decision to do something about it is in itself part of a social process. If there is a selection and definitional process then focussing solely on reasons for deviation (the study of etiology) and the reasons for not seeking treatment (the study of delay) and ignoring what constitutes a deviation in the eyes of an individual and his reasons for action may obscure important aspects of our understanding and eventually our philosophy of the treatment and control of illness.

Finally, this is not meant to be an essay on the importance of sociological factors in disease, but rather the presentation of an approach to the study of health and illness. Rather than being a narrow and limited concept, health and illness are on the contrary empirically quite elastic. In short, it is not merely that health and illness have sociological aspects, for they have many aspects, but really that there is a sense in which health and illness are social phenomena.

PART VI

Doctors and patients

15 The patient's offers and the doctor's responses

Michael Balint*

[*This reading is extracted from two chapters of a book developing the idea that inappropriate doctor responses to the patient's offer can lead to an (iatrogenic) illness. The data were gathered in the course of a highly structured series of group discussions extending over several years. All the available details of a case would be examined and subjected to searching questioning by the doctors in the group. Cases were followed up from time to time. The data are non-systematic in the sense that there was no formal sampling of cases in general practice and so we cannot be clear as to how frequently the kinds of problems described occur. The extract concentrates on problems that arise in doctor-patient relationships but the reader should be aware that elsewhere in the book and in subsequent publications (Balint and Balint 1961; Balint et al. 1966; Balint et al. 1970; Balint, E. and Norrell 1973) the helpful use of specialist examinations and consultations is considered. The author was a distinguished British psychoanalyst and doctor.*]

Let us take a rather simple case, one well known to every practitioner. Dr E. in charge of Case 5 reported in June 1954:

Case 5

Mr U., aged thirty-six. A highly-skilled workman, earning about £15 per week, married, two children. Very happy, apart from the fact that the younger boy, four years ago, had acute nephritis, and has been rather ill ever since. Mr U. had polio when a child and his left leg is about four inches shorter, requiring a boot. He deals with his infirmity extremely well, however. The boy's illness is rather tragic, but he copes with it quite well, although the illness gets his wife down. He runs a car, and takes his family out for weekends.

* extracted from M. Balint, *The Doctor, His Patient and the Illness* (1957) London: Pitman: 21–6, 69–75

In February while he was at work someone tampered with an electric connection and he got a very severe shock. He was thrown clear, but was out for about fifteen minutes. He came round and recovered completely. I think he then saw the doctor at the works or perhaps they sent him to the casualty department of the local hospital. Two or three weeks ago he came to see me, complaining of pains all over the front of his chest, the lower part of his back, right leg, and right hand, and saying that the pains were getting worse and worse. I examined him thoroughly and came to the conclusion that no organic damage had been done, although he thought that something had happened to him through the electric shock. As he seemed rather worried about it, I suggested that I get a specialist's opinion, which he accepted. He came to see me last night. He had had all the examinations. The letter to me from the hospital said that they could not find anything, and that 'we would like the patient to be seen by our psychiatrist'. I told him that nothing wrong had been found, and he said that was funny because his pains were much worse. He said, 'They seem to think I am imagining things – I know what I have got.' After talking a few minutes in a very pleasant manner, he said he thought the hospital might have made a mistake. He is definitely ill, and would like to know what condition he could have causing all these pains. 'What does the book say about it?' I did not answer, except to say that it was not a matter of looking up the books, that, for example, if he had a broken leg he would not ask me the cause of it, but would ask me to get it better. Finally I said that as he could not accept the view of the hospital, would he like to go to an entirely different hospital to be examined again? He was not keen, saying that they would do the same thing and would not find anything wrong. I was not sure how to get on, what was the next step, so I suggested that he should come back for further discussion in a week's time.

Let us start with the problem already mentioned: the patient 'proposing an illness' to the doctor – a very important first step in the history of any patient. In this case, in different periods, we can study an accepted compromise, an offer by the patient, then one by the doctor, the rejection of both of them in turn, and finally some of the ensuing consequences.

First, the accepted compromise. A severely handicapped man achieves, with the help of his understanding doctor, a highly satisfactory mental and physical equilibrium – very likely somewhat overpressing himself and overcompensating his physical shortcomings by high efficiency. Then, out of the blue, he is subjected to a severe electric shock, causing unconsciousness and possibly – in the psychological aspect – more than that. His reaction is a gradual development of pains in the whole front part of the body – the part which was facing in the direction from which the shock came – with the conspicuous exception of his damaged leg. The whole picture, i.e., the illness 'proposed', strongly suggests a psychological reaction – a queer mixture of fear, admission, and denial – as if he were saying, 'Something terrible has happened – I am afraid I have been badly damaged on my whole front, possibly my already disabled leg also; but no, that cannot be; I have pains practically everywhere except in my left leg'.

It is at this point that the doctor gets to work. Faithful to his training, he first sets out to exclude all possible physical complications, although there is no evidence to suggest any. After all, the accident happened in February and the patient did not come until the end of May. Still, the first move is to ask for a surgeon's opinion. As expected, this turns out to be negative, and the doctor's conscience about his responsibility is put at rest. He now tries to switch the patient to a second set of examinations, this time by a psychiatrist.

But what happened to the patient – and, still more important, in the patient – in the meantime? He came to his old trusted friend, the family doctor, prompted by pains, anxieties, fears, but otherwise in a trusting and friendly mood, hoping for help, understanding, and sympathy. It is true that he received a fair amount of all of them, but was then put through the mill of a routine hospital examination, almost certainly with a number of white-coated strangers firing searching questions at him. Perhaps he did, perhaps he did not, realize that everybody was getting more and more concerned about a possible claim for compensation, or to use a more fashionable term, about a possible compensation neurosis, and trying their best to prevent him from sliding into it. What he certainly did realize, however, was that all the doctors were at pains to convince him that *there was nothing wrong with him, i.e., they were rejecting his proposition.* When he came back to his doctor with the hospital report, the previous trusting, friendly attitude had been badly shaken, the model patient had turned into a disappointed, suspicious, mistrustful man.

In Mr U.'s case everything went satisfactorily until he was sent for a hospital examination. Previously the relationship between the patient and the doctor, in fact between the doctor and the whole family, had been excellent, although a good deal of strain had to be borne on both sides because of the grave illness of the younger boy. Not even the 'illness' provoked by the accident could upset the spirit of friendly cooperation. Only when the patient suspected that the doctors would somehow reject his 'propositions', i.e., either did not understand his illness or, still worse, did not care to understand it, did the relationship suffer. The patient started feeling – dimly at first – that perhaps the doctors were no longer on his side, that possibly they were actually against him. The hitherto model patient was thus forced first into an argument with his doctor, an argument which might later develop into a major battle. Yet we should not forget that despite this strain and suspicion the patient is still frightened and lost, desperately in need of help. His chief problem, which he cannot solve without help, is: what is his illness, the thing that has caused his pains and frightens him? In his own words, 'What does the book say?'

I wish to emphasize here that nearly always this is the chief and most immediate problem; *the request for a name for the illness, for a diagnosis*. It is only in the second instance that the patient asks for therapy, i.e., what can be done to alleviate his sufferings on the one hand, and the restrictions and deprivations caused by the illness, on the other.

Not paying attention to this order of importance is the cause of a very frequent form of irritation and of bitter disappointment in the doctor-patient relationship – another undesirable side-effect of the drug 'doctor'. When a patient, after a series of careful and conscientious examinations, is told that nothing is wrong with him, doctors expect that he will feel relieved and even improve. Admittedly this happens fairly often, but in quite a number of cases just the opposite occurs and the doctor's usual reaction to this – in spite of its frequency, always unexpected – event is pained surprise and indignation. This perhaps could be avoided if doctors would bear in mind that finding 'nothing wrong' is no answer to the patient's most burning demand for a name for his illness. Apart from the almost universal fear that what we have found is so frightening that we will not tell him, he feels that 'nothing wrong' means only that we have not found out and therefore cannot tell him what it is that frightens or worries him and causes him pain. Thus he feels let down, unable to explain and accept his pains, fears, and deprivations. It would certainly be no help to him to know that occasionally his suspicions are justified; that the statement 'nothing wrong' sometimes really means that medicine does not know what is wrong in his particular case.

The collusion of anonymity

In difficult cases, the general practitioner does not, as a rule, carry the burden of responsibility alone. Usually he asks and receives help from his specialists. The difficulties which prompt him to ask for help may be also described (viewed from a psychological angle) as crises of confidence. Either the doctor feels that he may not know enough to be able to help his patient, or the patient has doubts about the sufficiency of his doctor's knowledge and skill. The appearance of consultants introduces a number of new factors in the doctor-patient relationship. Let us again start with a case.

Mr K., when Dr Y. saw him, complained mainly of abdominal pains on and off; the pain often doubled him up and was followed by diarrhoea. He usually suffered severe pain before defaecation, sometimes the motion causing a burning sensation. In 1940 his former doctor sent him to see a surgeon, who suggested after due investigations that his trouble might be due to adhesions. He was given luminal and atropine.

In addition to all the symptoms mentioned above he complained of giddiness and added that he was afraid of crowds, going to the cinema, going to the barber to have his haircut. His clinical history was complicated through a fall, with a fracture of the spine, in 1939. Since then he also complained of twitching in his right leg, with prickly-heat sensations. This happened only at night.

Mr K. (in his doctor's words) visited me once or twice a week regularly over a long period. On clinical examination I could not find anything organically wrong that would justify his ill health. The search for psychological causes always led back to his dislike of his work. He always improved very quickly on sick leave.

In February 1951 I sent him back to the surgeon, who again could not find anything abnormal in his alimentary system. In June I sent him to Dr S., hoping for enlightenment from a psychiatric specialist. Mr K.'s symptoms persisted, and he sometimes felt near collapse even without pains. Once or twice he was taken to the casualty department of a nearby hospital. In October 1951 he attended the teaching hospital, where Dr S. is head of the Department of Psychological Medicine, for a narco-analytic session. I could never extract a report on this. He was, however, referred to the medical out-patients' department, where the possibility of gallstone was considered. I was rather shocked that this should have been overlooked all the time and might have been the cause of his symptoms. After further investigations he was operated on in January 1952. After his operation he was fit and entirely free of complaints until the middle of April. Then he returned to me with recurrence of spasm, diarrhoea, pain under left costal margin, giddiness. I tried to convince him that we had left no stone unturned, that now after the removal of his gallstones there could be no organic cause, that his symptoms were entirely due to psychological factors, that he had to overcome his anxieties and dislikes in order to cope with his problem. I did not give him any more medicine.

I saw him again two days ago. He was in a happily resigned mood. I went once more with him over his whole life, and this time tried to discuss also his sexual life. There seemed to be no clue at all, or probably I was not successful in overcoming his resistance.

I want to draw attention to an important point in this case. The doctor in charge was not alone. Being a careful man, time and again – as we learnt from his report – he referred his puzzling patient to various specialists. There were many of them, and in consequence there were many reports. As their spirit, their way of thinking, is most important for my argument, I propose to quote some of them. To give a coherent picture I have chosen all the reports of the dramatic period leading up to the operation, i.e., from February 1951 to March 1952.

Surgeon, writing from H. Hospital.   *23.2.1951*

Dear Dr Y.,

                                   Mr K.

Thank you for sending this patient to see me again. Gastroscopy shows a normal stomach apart from a small fine scar.
Barium enema shows a normal colon.
I have reassured him that there is no evidence of any growth. He is still overweight. I think he would be more comfortable on a light diet.

Psychiatrist, from his consulting rooms.   *5.6.1951*

Dear Dr Y.,

Yesterday I saw your patient Mr K. on your kind recommendation, for which many thanks.
I originally saw Mr K. on October 2, 1944, when he was complaining of cramps and tremors, and other symptoms which might have had a spinal origin. He had fallen on the ice and injured his back in 1939. X-ray revealed a fracture of the eleventh dorsal vertebra and he was four months in a plaster jacket in hospital. His cramps started in the right foot about seven months after the accident.
I formed the impression that he was an hysteric, but, in order to be on the safe side, especially as both ankle jerks were absent (they still are), I sent him to Dr Z. (a leading neurologist at J. Hospital). I never had a report from Dr Z., who I understand referred the patient to Dr I. at Y. Hospital.

Mr K. still complains of cramps, especially before going off to sleep, and more particularly in hot weather. He does not pay much attention to this symptom nowadays. His chief complaint of late is of pain in the right half of the abdomen ... In so far as his symptoms are consciously motivated, I think that they provide a 'cover' for his various failures in life; and I do not think that he is likely to be very responsive to psychotherapy of any kind.

However, I will have him registered at the Z. hospital and add his name to our psychotherapy waiting list, which, by the way, is fantastically long, as you might expect.

Physician in charge of Medical Out-patients, Z. Hospital. 30.11.1951

Dear Dr. Y.,

Re Mr K.

This patient was referred to me by Dr E. of the Department of Psychological Medicine on behalf of Dr S. He gives a history of abdominal pain coming in attacks, four of which have occurred in the last year, and are associated with pain in the right side of the stomach. He has no vomiting. The attacks last four to five hours and generally mean admission to a hospital. He volunteered the statement that the jolting of a bus worried him also.

On examination he looks fit, but has a dirty tongue. There was resistance of the upper abdomen, and two scars from an acute appendicitis associated with peritonitis, for which he was operated on in 1935. There was no obvious enlargement of the liver or gall bladder, no renal discomfort and he had not lost weight. I feel that he does require further investigation, but, as you know, X-rays are difficult at the present time. He states that he was X-rayed this year at the H. Hospital, [and given] a barium meal, and I would very much like you to send us a copy of the report they sent you. I feel that the possibility of gallstones must be excluded, but again there is the X-ray difficulty, and I would like to wait a period of three months. In the interval will you put him on Pil. Cholelith (Parke Davis & Co.,) the number controlled by his bowel motions, and I will review him again at the end of this time.

(Copy to Dr S.)

Physician, E. Hospital,   *16.12.1951*

Dear Dr Y.,

Re Mr K.

Many thanks for letting me see this patient. I think the reports from the various doctors are almost more interesting than the patient. I disagree with my illustrious colleagues at Z. as regards the absense of knee jerks. There is no doubt that they are present, but I could not elicit the ankle jerks beyond doubt. The Plantars are flexor. Babinski's sign is not present. This, together with normal abdominal reflexes and pupil reactions, can be taken as almost conclusive evidence against central or peripheral neurological pathology. He was vaguely tender in his abdomen, more on the right side, but certainly nothing decisive and localized. I could not convince myself of a tenderness over the gallbladder. P.R. I noticed a tender internal pile on the right side and an ampulla filled with spastic scybala.

The beginning of his trouble dates back to the time not long after his abdominal operations, and with this in mind I have asked for a barium meal and follow-through to clarify the picture as much as possible. If any medication is required it should be spasmolytics as it is already done. He might benefit from Vichy water tablets two to four times a day for ten days at a time.

Surgeon, E. Hospital.   *12.3.1952*

Dear Dr Y.,

Re Mr K.

I saw the above-named patient of yours again in the Out-patients Department on 10.3.52. he was an in-patient from 22.1.52 to 18.2.52. I removed his gall bladder and found chronic cholecystitis with gallstones. Convalescence was uneventful and he is now free of complaints. I have discharged him.

This case is a very good example of what we call the 'collusion of anonymity'. No one was really responsible for the decision to perform the operation. The first surgeon examined the patient conscientiously, but did not find anything, and fobbed him off with some 'reassurance' and a light diet. The patient then saw a psychiatrist privately who did another lot of physical examinations and, though not very confident about psychotherapy, put him on the waiting list. Next, the patient was, in due course, seen by the two chief assistants to the psychiatrist (these two did not write reports) was whisked off to a physician, and the suspicion of gallstones emerged. The doctor was ashamed of having missed the 'right' diagnosis, a second opinion was asked, the physician disagreeing with the psychiatrist but agreeing to the gallstones, and in consequence the patient's gall bladder was removed. The second surgeon is the last – proudly discharging the patient after operation, free of complaints. Nobody mentioned, and perhaps nobody was even interested in, what happened inside the patient while he was being whisked from doctor to doctor, eventually landing on the operating table.

16 The face-to-face interaction and after the consultation

Gerry Stimson & Barbara Webb*

[*This reading is extracted from a book describing a small-scale intensive study of general practice in Swansea, Wales. In the presentation of the research data the authors develop many insights into the nature of the doctor-patient consultation, demonstrating, as in the reading, that it is part of a much larger social relationship to illness and disease. The authors are sociologists working in the UK.*]

The study of the patient perspective must be undertaken within the assumption that he is as much a participant in the play as he is recipient or audience.

Hans O. Mauksch (1972: 27)

Two themes guide our analysis of the face-to-face consultation: strategies and negotiation. Essentially both actors (although we concentrate on the patient) are concerned with the same problem. This problem is effective self-presentation. As in all interaction, the conscious and unconscious presentation of the self affects the behaviour of the other and calls forth a reaction by the other.

In the consultation there is the problem of the outcome that is desired by both actors. People do not hand over all control and decision-making to the doctor merely by becoming patients. The presentation of the self can be used as a strategy. The aim of the strategies used by both patient and doctor is to attempt to control and direct the consultation along their own desired lines, to persuade the other to recognize or accept a particular perspective on, and orientation to, the problem that has been brought.

* extracted from G. Stimson, and B. Webb, *Going to See the Doctor* (1975) London: Routledge & Kegan Paul: 37–87

Seeing the consultation in terms of each actor trying to influence the other brings in the concept of negotiation. For, far from the outcome of the consultation being determined only by the problem that the patient brings and by the diagnosis of the doctor, the outcome is a result of the mutual interaction ...

Negotiation is a process. That patient and doctor both use strategies to influence each other does not mean that one or other is going to be successful. But the concept of negotiation means that we see the outcome as the result of their interaction and the strategies they have each adopted, rather than as determined solely by the facts that are brought and the application of the skills that the doctor has.

The consultation does not take place in a vacuum. Both doctor and patient may have met before and will have foreknowledge of each other. This allows the patient to anticipate the consultation and rehearse strategies. Where the doctor and illness condition are well known and the patient feels certain of the encounter and able to predict its probable course, we suggest that presentation and control strategies may have less of a persuasive content and the effort may be concentrated on reinforcing a common understanding and on following the usual pattern of activity. The most obvious example of this is the repeat prescription regime, which Marinker (1970) refers to as the 'truce', where a pattern of consultation has become routine. Yet negotiation does not cease; the inference is that reinforcement is necessary in order to ensure the continuation of such relations.

Of course it may be the case that the approach of the doctor is well known but the patient is dissatisfied with that approach. For example, a doctor may tend to treat many conditions with his 'favourite drug' and the patient may desire some other form of treatment. Or he may be predisposed to certain actions: '[He is known as] Doctor Undress – he makes you strip to the waist and that's only when you've got a sore throat, and he is very partial to internals for everything you have.' The patient may feel this behaviour is inappropriate and tactics may then be used by the patient to dissuade the doctor from his usual routine.

Although strategies may be planned through the patient having prior expectations of the encounter and having anticipated the problematic aspects of communication, they may also develop in the course of the interaction. This emphasizes the emergent and negotiable features of the interaction.

In emphasizing the negotiable aspects of the consultation, however, we do not pretend that the strategies are enacted in an open area. There are several limits on the possibilities for action. First, there is the limitation on the interaction imposed by the organization of medical care in the UK. The patient usually sees just one doctor for primary medical care and has limited ability to change doctors. It is consequently difficult for the patient to push disagreement with a doctor to the level of open conflict. The patient is very often in a position of 'take it or leave it'. Second, the patient is somewhat limited in his possibilities for action in that he perceives his knowledge, and the information available to him, to be of a different order from that of the professional.

A third limit is in the actors' perceptions of what is possible. Thus, patients may perceive that they are constrained by the amount of time available for the consultation, or they may feel constrained because the interaction takes place on the doctor's territory.

The fourth limitation to the strategic interaction concerns areas of implicit agreement in interaction. Order in the consultation is maintained by complicity, by agreements on the way certain aspects of the encounter are to be managed: such things as the use of jokes, the modes of address each use, the emotional flatness of the consultation, and the use of reassurance and empathy. Such aspects might, in lay terms, be summed up as 'good manners'.

What it is important to realize with these limitations to negotiation is not that the above are not all negotiable – for example, the patient *can* insist that the doctor devotes more time to the problem – but that they are *less* negotiable than other aspects of the consultation.

Presenting a problem to the doctor

In discussing the patient's prognosis in the consultation, a report from a working party of the Royal College of General Practitioners (1972) advises the doctor to ask himself certain questions:

> 'What must I tell this patient? How much of what I learned about him should he know? What words shall I use to convey this information? How much of what I propose to tell him will he understand? How will he react? How much of my advice will he take? What degree of pressure am I entitled to apply?' (p. 17)

If we change the second from last of these questions to read, 'How much notice will he take of what I say?' then these could be exactly the questions that the patient poses to himself when seeing the doctor. For the patient considers, both prior to and during the consultation, *what to say* to the doctor. Under this heading we deal with the patient's interpretation and selection of facts and the ways in which he attempts to put these across to the doctor with the maximum effect.

In perceiving his symptoms, the patient attempts to *interpret* them, and in explaining these symptoms both to himself and to the doctor, he is defining, categorizing, and causally linking them to other factors which he feels may be related. For example, the disorder may be presented in conjunction with another physical condition that the patient believes to be relevant. One woman explained her problem to the doctor in this way: 'I've had a lot of headaches lately – I wondered if it could be anything to do with my blood pressure?' The symptoms may be described in terms of a social context which the patient sees as significant, e.g., the woman patient who told the doctor she believed her anxiety and 'nerves' stemmed from her worries about a delinquent daughter. This interpreting is partly an attempt at self-diagnosis and partly an attempt to 'put the doctor on the right lines'. What is significant to the patient may not be so for the doctor, who may dismiss the patient's perceptions and interpretations as having little relevance and may probe for other factors that the patient has not mentioned ...

As well as having to define or recognize a problem and putting this into words, the patient is also involved in 'figuring out' the doctor. Both parties are 'sizing each other up'. The patient may not agree with the doctor's interpretation of the symptoms, especially when this does not accord with his own preconceived ideas and the doctor has not stated his interpretation in terms sufficiently convincing to persuade the patient to accept it. One young woman, consulting the doctor about her small child whose problem the doctor had interpreted as being unimportant and 'nothing to worry about', persistently reiterated that the symptoms in her child were both unusual and worrying: 'Yes, but it's most unusual for him to keep vomiting up his feed like this. And as I say, he's never been like this before.' In cases such as this, the patient may make further and more obvious attempts to persuade the doctor to acknowledge her own perspective on the problem: 'I said, "Well, what about these dizzy spells I've been having doctor?"And he just sat back and stared at me blankly ... so to help him I said, "Could it be anything to do with my age?"'

From all the many and varied pieces of information that could be given, the patient has also to be *selective* in verbal presentation. This selection may be largely unconscious – in any communication the speaker is necessarily selective – or it may be consciously planned. The problem in selecting what to say is that of estimating what is relevant and significant and what it is necessary or expedient to verbalize.

Very often all information is not given at the outset, almost as though the patient is not sure what is relevant. During the course of the inter-action, the patient may select and introduce other topics in response to the doctor's own interpretation and approach to the problem. For example, at a late stage in the presentation of her daughter's symptoms, a mother said: 'She has had a lot of injections lately.' Although this was phrased as a statement rather than a question, it was offered in a way that seemed to raise the question of whether the injections could have had anything to do with the child's present symptoms. The patient may offer various facts, suggesting or hinting at a possible causal relationship. The patient may select information according to criteria he thinks the doctor wants or needs to hear (those aspects which are believed will have meaning for a doctor) and what he, the patient, wants to tell the doctor and thinks he should be told ...

The doctor, too, is selective in what he decides to tell the patient. The doctor may not inform the patient of the type of drug he is prescribing or of possible side effects of the treatment. Similarly, the patient may withhold from the doctor information that he feels will place him in a disadvantaged position, for example, an admission that he has not followed instructions or that he fears a course of action proposed by the doctor. A woman told the interviewer that she was 'terrified' of her forthcoming operation: '... but don't write that down. Don't tell the doctor I said that, he'd shout at me if he heard me say that.' ...

Influencing the doctor

The ways in which people present themselves in the surgery may be viewed as strategies influencing the course of the consultation. We do not claim that the patient or the doctor always consciously adopt strategies to influence each other. The desire to influence may only be implicit in the presentation. The way in which the facts are presented to the doctor is an expression of a certain approach on the part of the patient, whether this approach is a request for a sickness certificate, a desire that the doctor should give attention to symptoms that are seen to be a problem, or simply a desire that the doctor makes all the decisions. Verbal and non-verbal control strategies are attempts to put across and reinforce that approach. Likewise, the doctor attempts to influence the interaction along his own desired course. The doctor may have repeated his actions so often that they are generally performed at the level of routine and are not consciously invoked except when that routine is disrupted. For both, the strategies are part of a repertoire, to be invoked when the situation permits. The efforts made by each to influence the interaction give the consultation its bargaining quality.

In the following example from a surgery consultation, a patient is trying to persuade the doctor that her problem merits medical attention.

The woman patient presents her symptoms to the doctor. He can find no explanation for them in the examination he makes or from the medical history on the patient's record card. As a position of stalemate is reached, the patient herself finally offers a proposed course of action in the light of the doctor's seeming inaction. She persists in offering the symptoms as a matter of concern and succeeds, by proposing a solution of her own, in gaining the doctor's recognition that some action should be taken. The consultation began with the woman describing 'odd pains' and giddiness and complaining that she had put on weight. We begin the dialogue with her speaking while the doctor examines her.

Patient: I've taken tablets. I thought I could fight it off.
Doctor: Mmm. Uh-huh.
Patient: This morning I couldn't even drink my cup of tea so I knew something was wrong.
Examination ends.
Doctor: Well, that's normal, there's nothing wrong there.
Patient: Well, I don't know what causes it, I'm sure.
Doctor: Your blood pressure's all right, there's nothing the matter there.
Patient: Nothing to worry about? Oh well, there you are then.
Doctor: Are you sure you've put on half a stone?
Patient: Definitely.
Pause in dialogue.
Patient: Is there something I could stop eating? I can't wear my clothes now.
Doctor: Cut out sugar in your tea and flour products, take them only in moderation. Try that and see how you go on. It'll take some time mind.
Patient (laughing): Oh I know that!
Both begin to joke about eating and weight problems.

There is rarely open conflict in the consultation. Both parties generally recognize and retain some semblance of formality and exercise restraint to prevent the encounter from completely 'breaking down'. A patient seldom makes accusations to a general practitioner's face about what are considered to be inefficiencies and inadequacies; similarly, a doctor rarely loses his temper with a patient. If it appears that this point is being approached, one actor seems to step down and attempts to avoid the issue or heal the breach. A patient who failed to keep her hospital appointment evoked the doctor's annoyance. During the consultation he said to her: 'Well I'm sorry, Betty. What do you expect me to do?

I've done as much as I can ... What's the use if you don't do anything I say?' Betty remained silent throughout, muttering her apologies just before leaving.

Verbal and non-verbal control strategies are often covert and rarely obvious or explicit. On the part of the patient they appear to operate beneath a façade of compliance and acquiescence. The thoughts of the patient which are not articulated during tense or difficult exchanges such as that above, may form the basis for 'stories' told about doctors when the patient is well away from the surgery ...

After the consultation

What happens after the patient has left the doctor's room? Our analysis of the consultation process continues beyond the face-to-face contact between patient and doctor. We see the process as including thoughts and conversations about the consultation, and the use of the treatment that has been prescribed by the doctor.

It is known from quantitative studies of patients' use of prescribed medicines, that a high proportion of patients do not follow the instructions of their doctors when taking prescribed medicines. If the treatment is a drug the patient may decide not to take the prescription to the pharmacist or may have it dispensed and not use the drug. The patient may begin to use the drug and then discontinue, or may use it with a frequency or in a dosage other than that advised by the doctor. Other types of treatment, too, may be used in ways other than those suggested by the doctor ...

Given that various processes – making sense of what happened, reappraisal, and evaluation – occur after the patient leaves the surgery, it becomes apparent that there is not necessarily any simple link between the doctor's action in prescribing a treatment, and whether or not, or in what way, that treatment is used by the patient. It is indeed difficult to divorce these processes from the patient's treatment decisions and actions.

An initial orientation towards the use of the treatment is found in the reappraisal and evaluation of the consultation. Patients may feel confused or be unable to make sense of exactly what happened, or be in some doubt over the nature of the treatment prescribed. They may decide to 'play safe' and do nothing, as in the case of an elderly woman who consulted her doctor over two recurrent problems – cystitis and blood pressure. She was given two sets of pills:

'When I got the tablets home, I didn't know which to take – the cystitis tablets for blood pressure, or the other tablets for cystitis when I got it, so I never took any. See what I mean? You get very confused.'

If, on the other hand, the patient is convinced on leaving the consultation that the doctor has not made a correct diagnosis, his prescribed treatment may be rejected. One woman, for example, felt that the doctor had failed to appreciate the 'real' nature of her complaint. She had complained of pain behind the eye, while he had given her ointment for the skin around the eye. She had then made an appointment on her own initiative to see an 'eye doctor' and explained: 'I haven't used the ointment because I didn't want it to affect what's really wrong with me.'...

Where do people get their ideas about the use of medicines? Seeing the patient in the formal setting of the consultation the doctor may be led to believe that he is the main source of people's ideas about medicines. He may be a source of ideas, but he is by no means the only source. On two occasions the researcher was asked for advice: on one occasion as to whether the prescribed pills were 'likely to do any good' and another time whether a proposed operation was 'a good idea – do you think I should have it done?'

Advice may be sought out, or may come almost fortuitously in everyday conversations about health and illness. Members of the family are obviously important in this respect. One woman in a group discussion described what happened after seeing the doctor:

'I'd just got back from the surgery when my mother phoned. I told her what he [the doctor] had given me, tranquillizers, and she said to me: "About these pills, you don't want to be drugged all the time; now when you feel better you stop taking them, all right?"'

Medication may be discussed with friends, as well as the family. Experiences may be compared, or the medication may be suggested as potentially useful to someone else. In one group discussion a woman and her friends described how they compared the tablets the doctor had prescribed for them, in order to 'see if we have the same things'. And another, recalling her last bout of bronchitis:

'The last time I went about bronchitis, he [the doctor] gave me these new pills. "Just come out", he said, and you know, they did work, they were better than the ones I had before. And so, there's this other lady I know also gets it badly, so I told her to tell the doctor to give her these ones.'

People have many sources of knowledge which contribute to their over-all perspective and actions with regard to the doctor's advice and instructions. 'I have learnt about diabetes – I have a sister who is a nurse', one male patient stated, and added that he had also 'read up' a good deal about his complaint in medical textbooks. Or the university student who said: 'In my experience I've found that they often don't give you the right treatment. Because I've worked in a chemist, I usually know what it is.'

The pharmacist is also a frequently-used source of ideas and influence relating to treatment decisions; patients will ask him to suggest some remedy before going to the doctor, or present him with a prescription from the doctor and ask his opinion on it.

This, then, is the broader setting in which evaluations of the doctor, reappraisals of the consultation, and treatment decisions and actions are taken. Local friendship and family networks make possible the exchange of information on what drugs are available, what they are to be used for, what the effects are, and how and when they should be taken or not taken. A person is unlikely simply to return from the doctor's surgery and take the treatment that has been prescribed. It is more likely that the doctor's action and the treatment will be discussed and evaluated. Medication decisions will be made in the light of these discussions, in the light of the person's experiences with the treatment, and in the light of past experiences with the doctor and other illnesses and treatments.

Our argument and illustrations have been mainly connected with one type of prescribed treatment – drugs – which is the most common treatment in general practice. In outlining the processes and influences, our argument may be as applicable to other treatments and also to notions of illness and decisions to consult. People live their problems and illnesses socially; they cannot be viewed as isolated individuals responding automatically to the instructions of their doctors.

This brings us to the crucial paradox of general practice: while the patient's ability to control the outcome of the consultation is limited, he has considerable ability to control what happens after he has left the doctor's presence. In the consultation, the doctor makes the treatment decisions; after the consultation, decision-making lies with the patient.

17 Uncertainty in medical prognosis: clinical and functional

Fred Davis*

[This paper has been reduced from the original by only a small amount in accordance with the editors' general strategy. The author is Professor of Sociology in the USA.]

Medical sociology is indebted to Talcott Parsons for having called attention to the important influence of uncertainty on the relationship between doctor and patient in the treatment of illness and disease (Parsons 1951). This is described as a primary source of strain in the physician's role, not only because clinically it so often obscures and vitiates definitive diagnoses and prognoses, but also because in an optimistic and solution-demanding culture such as ours it poses serious and delicate problems in the communicating of the unknown and the problematic to the patient and his family. In line with this view, Renee Fox has recently made an insightful analysis of the curriculum of a medical school, showing how, both from a formal and an informal standpoint, one of its functions is to socialize the student to cope more successfully with uncertainty (Fox 1957).

Granting the self-evident plausibility of the hypothesis, sociological

* extracted from the *American Journal of Sociology* (1960) 66: 41–7, July

studies of medical practice thus far have neglected to assess empirically its scope and significance in the actual treatment of specific illnesses or diseases. As a ready-made explanation of a disturbing element in the relationship between doctor and patient, the concept uncertainty stands in danger of being applied in a catch-all fashion whenever, for example, the sociologist notes that communication from doctor to patient is characterized by duplicity, evasion, or other forms of strain. That other factors having relatively little to do with uncertainty can also systematically generate strain in the relationship may unfortunately be ignored because of the disposition to subsume phenomena under pre-existent categories.

The present paper examines the scope and significance of uncertainty as evidenced in the treatment of a particular disease. Specifically, it seeks to distinguish between 'real' uncertainty as a clinical and scientific phenomenon and the uses to which uncertainty – real or pretended, 'functional' uncertainty – lends itself in the management of patients and their families by hospital physicians and other treatment personnel. By extrapolation, this distinction suggests a fourfold typology of patterns of communication from doctor to patient analysis of which highlights important sources of strain other than uncertainty.

The disease in question is paralytic poliomyelitis, and the subjects are fourteen Baltimore families, in each of which a young child had contracted the disease. These were studied longitudinally over a two-year period by an inter-disciplinary team of social scientists and research physicians whose broad interest was in assessing the total impact of the experience on child and family. Except for one family that dropped out midway in the study, in each case the child with polio and his parents were interviewed at intervals from the time of the child's admission to a pediatrics ward in the acute stage of the disease to approximately a year and a half following his discharge from a convalescent hospital.

From the very first interview with the parents, held within a week or so following the child's admission to the hospital, to the fourteenth and final interview with them some two years later, the research (which also included direct observation) was aimed at determining at every stage what the parents knew and understood about polio in general and their child's condition in particular and through whom and how they came to acquire such knowledge and understanding as they had on these matters.

By bringing together the interview and observational data gathered from these several sources, it was possible to compare and contrast, at successive stages of the disease and its treatment, what the parents knew and understood of the child's condition with what the doctors knew and understood. One must assume that the doctor's knowledge of the disease and its physical effects is more accurate, comprehensive, and profound than that of the parents. The problem, then, could be stated: How much information was communicated to the parents? How was it communicated? And what consequences did this communication have on the parents' expectations of the child's illness and prospects for recovery? (Davis 1956). And, since in paralytic poliomyelitis (as in many other diseases and illnesses) uncertainty does affect the making of diagnoses and prognoses, an attempt was made to assess the scope, significance, and duration of uncertainty for the doctor. This then provided some basis for inferring the extent to which the parents' knowledge and expectations, or lack thereof, could also be attributed ultimately to uncertainty.

Now the pathological course of paralytic poliomyelitis is such that, during the first weeks following onset, it is difficult in most cases for even the most skilled diagnostician to make anything like a definite prognosis of probable residual impairment and functional disability. During the acute phase of the disease and for a period thereafter, the examining physician has no practical way of directly measuring or indirectly inferring the amount of permanent damage or destruction sustained by the horn cells of the spinal cord as a result of the viral attack. (It is basically the condition of these cells, and not that of the muscles neurologically activated by them, that accounts for the paralysis.) Roughly, a one- to three-month period for spontaneous recovery of the damaged spinal cells – a highly unpredictable matter in itself – must first be allowed for before the effects of the disease are sufficiently stabilized to permit a clinically well-founded prognosis.

During this initial period of the child's hospitalization, the physician is hardly ever able to tell the parents anything definite about the child's prospects of regaining lost muscular function. In view of the very real uncertainty, to attempt to do so would indeed be hazardous. To the parents' insistent question 'How will he come out of it?', the invariable response of treatment personnel was that they did not know and that only time would tell. Thus, during these first weeks the parents came to adopt a longer time perspective and more qualified outlook than they had to begin with (Davis 1956).

By about the sixth week to the third month following onset of the disease, however, the orthopedist and physiotherapist are in position to make reasonably sound prognoses of the amount and type of residual handicap. This is done on the basis of periodic muscle examinations from which the amount and rate of return of affected muscular capacity is plotted.

By this time, the element of clinical uncertainty regarding outcome, so conspicuously present when the child is first stricken, is greatly reduced for the physician, if not altogether eliminated. Was there then a commensurate gain in the parents' understanding of the child's condition after this six-week to three-month period had passed? Did they then, as did the doctors, come to view certain outcomes as highly probable and others as improbable?

On the basis of intensive and repeated interviewing of the parents over a two-year period, the answer to these questions is that, except for one case in which the muscle check pointed clearly to full re-covery, the parents were neither told nor explicitly prepared by the treat-ment personnel to expect an outcome significantly different from that which they understandably hoped for, namely, a complete and natural recovery for the child. This does not imply that the doctors issued falsely optimistic prognoses or that, through indirection and other subtleties, they sought to encourage the parents to expect more by way of recovery than was possible. Rather, what typically transpired was that the parents were kept in the dark. The doctors' answers to their questions were couched for the most part in such hedging, evasive, or unintelligibly technical terms (Kutner 1958) as to cause them, from many such contacts, to expect a more favourable recovery than could be justified by the facts then known. As one treatment-staff member put it, 'We try not to tell them too much. It's better if they find out for themselves in a natural sort of way.'

Indeed, it was disheartening to note how, for many of the parents, 'the natural way' consisted of a painfully slow and prolonged dwindling of expectations for a complete and natural recovery. This is ironical when one considers that as early as two to three months following onset the doctors and physiotherapists were able to tell members of the research team with considerable confidence that one child would require bracing for an indefinite period; that another would never walk with a normal gait; that a third would require a bone-fusion operation before he would be able to hold himself erect; and so on. By contrast, the parents of these children came to know these prognoses much later, if at all. And even then their understanding of them was in most instances partial and subject to considerable distortion.

But what is of special interest here is the way in which uncertainty, a *real* factor in the early diagnosis and treatment of the paralyzed child, came more and more to serve the purely managerial ends of the treatment personnel in their interaction with parents. Long after the doctor himself was no longer in doubt about the outcome, the perpetuation of un-certainty in doctor-to-family communication, although perhaps neither premeditated nor intended, can nonetheless best be understood in terms of its functions in the treatment system. These are several, and closely connected.

Foremost is the way in which the pretense of uncertainty as to outcome serves to reduce materially the expenditure of additional time, effort, and involvement which a frank and straightforward prognosis to the family might entail. The doctor implicitly recognizes that, were he to tell the family that the child would remain crippled or otherwise impaired to some significant extent, he would easily become embroiled in much more than a simple, factual medical prognosis. Presenting so unwelcome a prospect is bound to meet with a strong – and, according to many of the treatment personnel, 'unmanageable' – emotional reaction from parents; among other things, it so threatens basic life values which they cherish for the child, such as physical attractiveness, vocational achievement, a good marriage, and, perhaps most of all, his being perceived and responded to in society as 'normal, like everyone else'. Moreover, to the extent to which the doctor feels some professional compunction to so inform the parents, the bustling, time-conscious work milieu of the hospital supports him in the convenient rationalization that, even were he to take the trouble, the family could not or would not understand what he had to tell them anyway (Kutner 1958). Therefore, in hedging, being evasive, equivocating, and cutting short his contact with the parents, the doctor was able to avoid 'scenes' with them and having to explain to and comfort them, tasks, at least in the hospital, often viewed as onerous and time consuming.

Second, since the parents had been told repeatedly during the first weeks of the child's illness that the outcome was subject to great un-certainty, it was not difficult for them, once having accepted the idea, to maintain and even to exaggerate it, particularly in those cases in which the child's progress fell short of full recovery. For, equivocally, uncer-tainty can be grounds for hope as well as despair; and when, for example, after six months of convalescence the child returned home crippled, the parents could and characteristically did interpret uncertainty to mean that he still stood a good chance of making a full and natural recovery in the indefinite future. The belief in a recuperative moratorium was held long after there was any real possibility of the child's making a full recovery, and with a number of families it had the unfortunate effect of diverting them from taking full advantage of available rehabilitation procedures and therapies. In fact, with few exceptions the parents typically mistook rehabilitation for cure, and, because little was done to correct this misapprehension, they often passively consented to a regimen prescribed for the child which they might have rejected had they known that it had nothing to do with effecting a cure.

Last, it must be noted that in the art (as opposed to the science and technique) of medicine, a sociologically inescapable facet of treatment – often irrespective of how much is clinically known or unknown – is frequently that of somehow getting the patient and his family to accept, 'put up with', or 'make the best of' the socially and physically disadvantageous consequences of illness. Both patient and family are understandably reluctant to do this at first, if for no other reason than that it usually entails a dramatic revaluation in identity and self conception.

Clearly, then, clinical uncertainty is not responsible for all that is not communicated to the patient and his family. Other factors, interests, and circumstances intrude in the rendering of medical prognoses, with the result that what the patient is told is uncertain and problematic may often not be so at all. And, conversely, what he is made to feel is quite certain may actually be highly uncertain. As the rough fourfold schema of *Figure 7* suggests, there are at least two modes of communication (*2* and *3*) that reveal a discrepancy between what the doctor knows and what he tells the patient. Before turning to these, however, we shall consider the two 'pure', non-discrepant modes (*1* and *4*).

The first of these, 'communication' (*1*), refers to the common occurrence in which the physician can, in accordance with the state of medical knowledge and his own skill, make a reasonably definite prognosis of the condition requiring treatment and communicate it to the patient in terms sufficiently comprehensible to him. Though not always as uncomplicated as it sounds, this is perhaps the main kind of exchange of information between doctors and patients, particularly as regards the simple and minor ailments brought daily to the average practitioner's attention. It is also, of course, the ideal mode of communication towards which the relationship of doctor and patient universally aspires.

On the other hand, an 'admission of uncertainty' (*4*), where no other prognosis is clinically justifiable, is by its nature a more difficult and unstable mode of communication, the manifestations of which will vary considerably, depending on the personal and institutional contexts of practice. Such instability derives mainly from certain mutually reinforcing interests of the two parties: the doctor, who as a matter of professional obligation seeks to narrow the range of uncertainty as far as possible, and the patient, who wishes simply and often naively to know what is wrong and how he can be made to feel better. These and other pressures that would prevent an open admission of uncertainty can more easily be resisted in the bureaucratized hospital setting – as, indeed, they initially were in the case of the families of children with

	certainty	uncertainty
prognosis given patient	(1) communication	(2) dissimulation
prognosis not given patient	(3) evasion	(4) admission of uncertainty

Figure 7

polio – than, for example, in neighborhood private practice. For, given the widespread intolerance of uncertainty in our culture, the hospital-anchored physician is better insulated from the prejudices, sensitivities, and economic sanctions of those he treats than is his neighborhood counterpart (Freidson 1960).

Owing in large part to a currently inadequate scientific grounding, certain fields of medical practice, such as psychiatry, permit little more than admissions of uncertainty in a very large number of cases. Yet, even here, it is to be questioned whether the office psychiatrist can as a matter of course adopt the same unyielding, non-committal, anti-prognostic stance with his private, fee-paying patients as does the state-hospital psychiatrist with the severely mentally ill and their families – this despite the fact that nowadays, as with pneumonia and the common cold, the psychopathology treated in the mental hospital affords better grounds for prognosis than do the psychoneuroses and character disorders seen in the consulting room.

As these remarks imply, 'dissimulation' (2) – the rendering of a prognosis which the physician knows to be unsubstantiated clinically – is the more likely if the doctor's reputation and livelihood are derived for the most part from the favorable opinions and referrals of an independent lay clientele. Sheer professional vanity may, of course, also enter into it. The subtleties, ruses, and deceptions that betoken dissimulation, from the innocuous sugar-pill placebo to unwarranted major surgery, are too many and too imaginatively varied to consider here.

'Evasion' (3) – the failure to communicate a clinically substantiated prognosis – has already been considered at some length. As noted, this was the primary mode of communication employed by the hospital treatment staff when confronted with the queries and concerns of the parents. Little need be added here except to emphasize that the informal institutionalization of this mode is closely related to the practitioner's ability to remove himself from the many 'technically secondary' (i.e., non-organic) problems and issues that often follow in the wake of serious illness in the family. The large hospital, with its complex proliferation of specialized services and personnel, is particularly conducive to it, especially if the attending physician is not the patient's own but someone assigned to him.

18 Vocabularies of realism in professional socialization

Joan Stelling & Rue Bucher*

[*This paper has been reduced from the original by only a small amount in accordance with the editors' general strategy. The authors are Professors of Sociology in Canada and the USA, respectively.*]

... These data are drawn from a longitudinal study of professional socialization. All of the trainees entering two quite different training programmes in psychiatry during 1965, and all of the trainees entering a residency in internal medicine during 1965 and 1966 are the subjects of this study. We interviewed them when they first arrived and subsequently re-interviewed them at the end of each year. All of these in-depth interviews were tape-recorded. Three years of training were required for each specialty, although many of the internal medicine residents and a few of the psychiatry residents took a fourth year of sub-specialty training. In between interviews, we did participant observation to the degree necessary to give us an understanding of the situations in which the respondents were functioning. In addition, we interviewed a sample of the staff in each program, including both those who were full time and heavily involved in the training programs and those who were part time or voluntary. The numbers of entering residents were seven and

* extracted from *Social Science and Medicine* (1973), 7: 661–75

twenty-one for the two psychiatry programs, and fifteen in internal medicine. For this paper, we selected only those respondents with whom we had at least three interviews, so that the total number of respondents reported here is thirty-six ...

Mistakes

Our respondents were highly articulate people. They could express themselves clearly, in as much depth as they wished, and communicate with interviewers who were relative strangers to their world. One of the striking things about the interviews is how many of these articulate people suddenly became inarticulate when confronted with words like 'failure' and 'mistake'. Several persons simply told us, as their first response to the probes, that these words did not fit into their frame of reference ... Respondents began to fumble, pause at length, to make a number of false starts, parts of sentences, even sentences that were illogical or nonsensical. The transcription of recorded interviews tends to even out much of the false starts and incoherence of actual human speech. But all of our typists, without anything being said, on our part, put in more false starts, the 'uhs' and 'ahs', the pauses, and so forth, when they came to this material on the tapes. It was that strikingly different from the other materials. Here is a 'classic' instance of sudden incoherence:

I: 'What constitutes a failure in internal medicine?'
R: (relatively long pause) 'Probably just when a mistake is made.'
I: 'Do you know when a mistake is made – can you tell?'
R: 'Not right away, perhaps, but I think most of the time you can – a large proportion of the time you may say, gee, I wonder if I did wrong – you may not be sure. I don't – I don't think that's a mistake. I don't think that's a failure. Um, yes, doctors learn from the death of patients – no question about that. Now do they *cause* the death of patients – I suppose that's a failure. If a doctor causes the death of a patient and he knows it. Now, if he's not sure, that's not a failure, that's an experience, a learning experience'. . .

A minority of respondents, with more or less fumbling, did proceed to describe what they considered mistakes. But the fact that they could not respond to the words failure and mistake until they had *translated them into their own frame of reference* is a strong indication that these are lay, rather than professional, concepts.

So what were mistakes to these respondents? For both internists and psychiatrists if there was such a thing as mistakes, it was a matter of the wrong behavior when *any well-trained person ought to know better*. Furthermore, mistakes were about matters of *procedure and process*. Mistakes were never determined by outcomes. The language internal medicine residents used was significant. Mistakes were 'gross errors', 'obvious', and 'clear-cut mistakes'...:

> **I:** 'We were talking about knowing when you are in trouble. How do you differentiate between making a mistake and something that couldn't be helped?'
>
> **R:** 'By yourself?'
>
> **I:** 'Can you do it by yourself might be a good question, too.'
>
> **R:** 'Gee, I don't know if you can do it by yourself. That varies depending on the problem. You know, some things are clear-cut and you've made a mistake when you're finished. If you put a test tube into somebody to draw off a certain amount of ... and you put it in an artery and you get blood back it's quite evident you made a mistake, you know, and you may learn from it how to approach the procedure differently next time. Whereas you see a patient with a pain in his chest and you decide it's not coronary and he dies two hours later, you're never sure.'...

This respondent illustrates how, having indicated the type of thing that might be regarded as a mistake, a gross error, or a clear-cut mis-management of a technique, he begins to get into areas where it is not so obvious or clear cut. The following case bears upon the respondent's conception of things which physicians ought to know:

> 'I mean, you can, by laboratory determinations, pick up an anemia. Now some physicians still can't handle this correctly, and there's a failure of content of knowledge, I think. But you don't really have to know everything about an area to know that this is where the patient's trouble lies, and to know where to go for help, or where to direct the patient for further work on this sort of thing ...'...

Vocabularies of realism

In general parlance, the old quip that 'the operation was successful, but the patient died' precisely illustrates the difference between lay and professional perspectives. The layman is concerned with the results, the professional is focussed upon the work itself. The residents in both psychiatry and internal medicine began to evaluate their work in terms of doing the job, rather than in terms of the outcomes of their work. Furthermore, the language which they developed to evaluate their efforts was remarkably similar across these three groups of residents. There are two major themes in these vocabularies. The first basic theme, we will call the 'doing-one's-best' vocabulary. The second we can call the 'recognition-of-limitations' vocabulary. There is a third, more minor theme, which might be named 'gray areas', or indeterminacy. Let us, with ample quotations, illustrate the dimensions of these vocabularies.

Doing one's best

The 'doing-one's-best' vocabulary is particularly striking because it so sharply contrasts with the lay perspective. Knowing full well from their own experience that things do not always go well for patients, the respondents placed emphasis on whether they had done their best by the patient. If they have done their best they may feel sad, but not devastated by a bad outcome. The following quotation illustrates a psychiatry resident moving into this vocabulary. At the end of his first year of training, in the context of a discussion of outstanding experiences that occurred during the year ... he had begun to assimilate the idea that if the outcome of his work with a patient was not successful – i.e., if the patient committed suicide anyway – this was not necessarily indicative of a failure on his part. Two years later, upon completion of the residency programme, he articulated this theme far more clearly and succinctly:

'... the idea that I should do my job to the best of my ability and that didn't necessarily mean that I should feel guilty if the patient didn't get better ... some people criticize us for being hard-hearted in our views and say, "How can you possibly divorce yourself from the outcome of your work", and what they fail to realize is my work has to do not so much with the results, but has to do with the process. That's a revolutionary new idea, because what it means is it frees you, you know ... I admit that I'm much happier when my patients succeed and do better – but I think ... it frees you from the kind of guilty ruminations and feeling responsible for patients' behavior, which can effectively thwart any therapeutic effort.'

While not all the residents are so articulate, the idea that their culpability lies in whether or not they do their best, rather than in the results of their efforts, is frequently expressed. A psychiatry resident phrased it as follows:

'... you have an idea of what you think will work and what you don't ... what won't work for a certain kind of problem, whatever it is, you know. If you do the things you think will work and they don't that's not a failure, you know, you've done what you thought was best, and still it didn't work. It's a failure in the sense that you still have a problem, but it's not your failure. Ah, in other words, you don't have to be able to solve every problem that comes to – you have to be able to do what you think is best – and you have to do it.'

A part of the 'doing-one's-best' vocabulary is the concept of '*acceptable errors of judgement*'. Implicit in the previous quotations – and explicitly stated by some of the residents – is the recognition that doing one's best does not rule out the possibility of making a decision which subsequently turns out to have been wrong. However, if the wrong decision was appropriate, *given the circumstances in which it was made*, it is considered an acceptable error of judgement. An acceptable error is doing one's best with the information available at the time. One has to take action under particular circumstances, and these circumstances may lead one to make the wrong decision ...

For the medicine residents the acceptable errors are in situations in which the case is an extremely difficult one and in which other internists would have made the same decision or would have been equally unable to be sure of the correct decision or diagnosis. As one of the residents put it:

'Well, I think – ah – it's – ah – *you* may feel, I think, that – and there have been times when I felt – "I think I've – I've – I've harmed this patient. I've done something wrong." And yet, if you talk with other people they say, you know – they may not find fault with what you did at all ... you know, it was a judgement area. That what you did – if you took a hundred physicians you know, maybe half or more may have done exactly the same thing in your position.'

This example manifests the common theme that given the same set of circumstances anybody else would have done the same thing, and hence, that one could not have been expected to do otherwise. Thus, if an error was made, it was acceptable, or at least unavoidable.

Although the residents do not use the word, many of these examples imply that there is an element of luck involved: Whatever else, you do your best, and you win some and lose some. As one of the medicine residents says, 'Everybody has his coups ... and everybody has a few disasters'.

Recognition of limitations

Recognition of limitations refers to the concepts which these residents hold concerning the extent and ways in which patients can be helped ... The limitations are seen as those of the *field*, rather than any sort of personal inadequacy. When asked 'How much can medicine help people?', the medicine residents tend to respond in terms of limitations – how little internal medicine could help or how many patients there were that it could not help. They pointed out that if 'to help' meant 'to cure', as they apparently assumed it did to the layperson, then it could help very little. But they went on to indicate how medicine could help, in terms of *their* definitions of 'to help'. One of the residents gave a clear indication of his perception of this difference between the layperson and the professional:

> I: 'How much can you do for patients in internal medicine?'
> R: 'Less than the general public thinks but a moderate amount. Er, it depends very much on the patient. It's hard to answer that – there are some patients which you can do a great deal for ... if you mean how much can you do by diagnosing the patient and sending them on to the proper surgeons, then quite a bit.' ...

Note that if what is meant is to diagnose and refer to the proper person – acts which are the heart and soul of internal medicine to most of the residents in our sample – medicine can do 'quite a bit'. While this resident says, in effect, that the help lies in diagnosis and referral, others put the emphasis on mitigating the effects of disease; they talk about how few diseases they can cure or how few lives they can save, saying that what they can do is 'maintain the status quo', or prolong the patient's 'productive or functional life' ...

Gray areas

Another vocabulary prevalent among the medicine residents, but not in psychiatry, is that of 'gray areas' or judgement areas – situations in which there is more than one way of approaching and dealing with a problem and no clear guidelines for determining which of them, if any, is the best way. In other words, there are differing, but equally legitimate or justifiable, ways of working with a problem. In the words of one of the graduating residents:

> 'You get to see two or three different doctors approach a problem, and you soon understand that there is perhaps no one way or one

right way; I think that also makes you a lot more humble to see that there are several different ways to approach a problem and that patients will get better by some other way and not only your own way.'

After telling the interviewer that in most cases it was possible to distinguish mistakes, another resident continued:

'But there, I mean there *are* gray zones where it does become a matter of judgement. And although, you know, two decisions – or two different decisions could be made on certain problems, and only one, you know, one *can* be – one is chosen and may turn out to be wrong, and then you may think, "Well, what would have happened then?"'

Other residents emphasized that gray areas in medicine are the rule, rather than the exception, saying things like: 'There is no real black and white ... everything's gray,' and, '... there are no rights and wrongs. There are no blacks and whites. But I guess the more you – and the further you go on, the wider the field of gray becomes – less black and less white.' They point out that support can be found in the medical literature for almost any position one wishes to take *vis-à-vis* a given problem ...

Conclusion

Collective ways of coping with mistakes and failures are likely to be particularly well developed in a profession which has both high risk and fateful consequences. This leads us to expect that vocabularies of realism may be especially well elaborated in the world of medicine. In spite of the explosive nature of contemporary advances in medical science, there remain many gaps in knowledge and many areas in which diagnosis and treatment are highly problematic. These uncertainties and gaps in knowledge are reflected in our respondents statements about 'gray areas' and 'limitations of the field' ...

... There are two ways in which these data are suggestive of factors which may work against internal professional controls. The first has to do with visibility. As Freidson points out, the idea of regulation or control over professional services presupposes some visibility of performance, and clinical medicine is not generally characterized by high visibility (Freidson 1970: 179–80) ... As trainees go through these socialization programs, they focus increasingly on the process of doing their work and decreasingly on the final outcomes or results of that work. In other words, what they come to see as important in evaluating professional performance are precisely those processes which are likely to have the least visibility to professional colleagues.

It should be noted that trainees acquire these vocabularies under rather special circumstances. Their work with patients is much more visible than in most conditions of medical practice. Furthermore, they are being coached in 'doing-one's-best': Supervisors or attending men are reviewing with them the *process* of diagnosis and treatment. Thus, these vocabularies of realism originate under conditions where they might be deemed appropriate. Nevertheless, the point remains that most of these trainees then carried this language with them into quite different circumstances of practice ...

The vocabularies reported here can also be seen as contributing to the lack of adequate internal professional control over the quality of medical care. Certainly, a language which emphasizes the criterion of 'doing one's best', the ambiguities of decision-making, and which virtually annihilates the concept of 'mistake', can hardly be construed as supportive or encouraging stringent application of internal controls and sanctions. Where so much is dependent on circumstances, and so much is uncertain and ambiguous – in terms of knowing both what decision to make and, subsequently, whether a different decision would have led to better results – it would perhaps not be surprising that results become subordinate to processes, nor that a medicine resident reports an increasing tolerance for the mistakes of other physicians. The language is more compatible with the development of an attitude of 'There but for chance go I', than a willingness to identify and censure errors of judgement ...

19   Forecast and follow-up: an investigation into the clinical, social, and mental factors determining the results of hospital treatment

A. Querido*

[This reading has been taken from a much longer original in accordance with the editors' general strategy. The discussion of the patient sample (demonstrated to be reasonably representative of a typically general hospital), and of the differential results by diagnostic condition and type of 'distress' (both shown to be unimportant), have been heavily reduced. The original argument involved a long and detailed statistical presentation which has here been abridged and somewhat altered with the permission of the author who was the first Professor of Social Medicine at the University of Amsterdam, Netherlands, but has now retired.]

The problem

Earlier studies (Querido, 1958; Weijel and Willemse, 1955; De Levita, 1958) indicate that many patients admitted to a general hospital may be burdened by stresses which may or may not be interwoven with the somatic illness but may well impede the chances of complete recovery and so diminish the effect of the labours of the hospital staff.

The question therefore arises whether the chances of recovery are better for patients unburdened by stresses than for patients who are bearing stresses they are unable to handle.

* extracted from the *British Journal of Preventive and Social Medicine* (1959) **13**: 33–49

Methods

Method of integrative assessment

The completion and assessment of the psycho-social case history was the task of a team of three (a general physician, a social worker, and a psychiatrist) working parallel to but independent from the ordinary hospital staff for the purpose of this investigation.

The general physician was a young man who filled the role of ward doctor or family physician. It was his duty to establish and to maintain the contact with the patient and to interpret to those in the hospital who decide the fate of the patient, his human as well as his medical history. The psycho-social case history was started within forty-eight hours of admission, and at the same time the general physician took note of the clinical findings. Next, the case was discussed by the team. In some instances it was possible at this early stage to reach an opinion concerning the presence of stress and its nature; in others either the social worker or the psychiatrist felt the need of more extensive data. These might be provided by the general physician, or the psychiatrist or social worker might make his own investigation. After the required data had been gathered the team met again and this time attempted to reach a definite conclusion. Previous history and the patient's behaviour in former difficulties, his attitude towards actual problems, and his subjective expressions were taken into account.

A decision did not rest upon the question whether stress was adjudged to be present but upon the question whether the patient was hampered by his problems. When it was decided that the patient was not able to handle his problems and was hampered or burdened by them, the team used the expression *distress*. When problems were mentioned by the patient but the team judged that he was able to manage them, the expression *stress* was used. In this article, therefore, 'distress' refers to social and/or psychic tensions too heavy for the patient to bear, while 'stress' refers to tensions which are satisfactorily integrated in the patient's life pattern. The term 'somatic' means that no distress could be found or that the somatic illness was so serious that it dominated the entire picture. The type of 'distress' was classified as follows: psychic only; psychosomatic; somatic with psychic parallel problems; somatic with social parallel problems; somatic with psychic and social problems.

Furthermore, the work of the team was observed by a psychologist, who followed its group dynamic action and studied the way in which its judgement came into being. In this way it was possible to prevent the judgement of the team being distorted by the domination of any one member.

If it be agreed that the team's assessment may be considered as an integrated evaluation of the patients' problems the questions to be answered may be stated simply as follows: (i) What is the value of integrated and clinical assessments in relation to the patients' condition in the follow-up? (ii) Does the integrated assessment contain specific elements, and if so, are these elements different from those which comprise the clinical prognosis?

Method of follow-up assessment

An attempt was made to visit the patient in his home six months after discharge. It was not always possible to keep exactly to this period, which in some cases extended to eighteen months, the average being seven months after discharge.

The follow-up investigation was carried out by a physician who knew the contents of the clinical case history, but was unaware of the psycho-social data and the team's assessment. In reaching a conclusion on the condition of the patient, objective data (behaviour, resuming of work) as well as subjective observations were taken into account. It was not intended that factors of stress should be examined again, and although it was sometimes unavoidable to touch on these subjects during the visits, these findings were never used to change the original assessment of the team. The doctor undertaking the follow-up was unaware of the conclusions of the team and the team was not told about his conclusions to avoid bias in the later stages of their work.

There was some difficulty in formulating the follow-up assessment. The term 'cured' could not be used, because it required a distinction to be made between anatomical, physiological, and functional cure, and between objective and subjective cure. For some time the term 'benefit' was used, but this was finally rejected because it seemed to imply a too direct causal relationship between hospital admission and the later condition of the patient. Finally the neutral terms 'satisfactory' and 'unsatisfactory' were chosen, and these are used in the rest of this paper. Cases were assessed as 'satisfactory' when the patient was: (a) free from any complaint; (b) suffering from typical residual complaints (pain in scar, etc.) only; (c) free from any complaint for a time but now showing sharply-defined symptoms which could not possibly be related to the illness for which he had been admitted to hospital.

The term 'unsatisfactory' was used for all other cases, in which the patient was: (a) free from complaints for some time but now experiencing a return of the former symptoms; (b) suffering from complaints equal to or worse than those experienced before admission; (c) slightly improved but substantially unchanged; (d) suffering from a recurrence, with or without a complaint-free period.

Clinical assessment

The general physician made a prognosis in consultation with the department physician in the light of the clinical case history. An attempt was made to estimate the patient's chances of recovery as accurately as possible (recovery in the sense of a return of well-being and a disappearance of the symptoms which had led to admission) having regard to the medical, technical, and somatic side of the problem. This assessment was meant to show how far the illness was reversible. The prognosis was recorded as 'favourable' or 'unfavourable'.

The various assessments to be compared may thus be designated as follows:

assessment	good	bad
(1) integrated	no stress or stress	distress
(2) clinical	favourable	unfavourable
(3) follow-up	satisfactory	unsatisfactory

A psycho-social case history was taken of about 2,200 patients, admitted to the Weesperplein Ziekenhuis in Amsterdam. No selection of patients was made. All patients who were admitted as from February 1, 1955 were investigated, with the following exceptions: patients younger than fifteen and older than sixty-five; patients who on admission were in poor condition, great pain, or obviously dying; patients who could be expected to remain only a very short time, for instance for tonsillectomies; and, when admissions were very frequent every other patient was excluded.

In 1,128 of the cases the clinical prognosis was favourable. In 871 of the 1,630 cases the team reached the conclusion that no particular distress was present; in 759 cases distress was found. There was no relationship between the occurrence of distress and the age or sex of the patients.

The follow-up showed that 817 patients were in a satisfactory condition and 813 in an unsatisfactory condition.

Comparison of clinical assessment and team assessment

A diagnosis might be regarded as a summary of the condition of the patient at a given moment; the integrated team assessment is also a summary of the type of distress from which the patient is suffering. Both assessments are in a sense 'forecasts'. When the elements on which diagnosis is based are given a dynamic character, a prognosis arises, and in the same way the designation 'no stress' or 'distress' is a forecast because it has an implication for the future. This investigation aims at testing both forecasts against the observations made at a follow-up examination.

Before the results of this comparison are discussed, it must be decided whether the two forecasts are identical, whether 'no stress' means the same as 'prognosis favourable', and 'distress' means the same as 'prognosis unfavourable'.

'No stress' represents the judgement of the team that no tensions and conflicts are present in the patient which he is unable to manage. In this situation his chances of recovery depend solely on his bodily condition, and if on somatic grounds the clinical forecast is 'favourable', the patient's prospects are good. In such cases 'prognosis favourable' and 'no stress' are identical, in the sense that they forecast the same result.

But if the clinical prognosis is 'unfavourable', the team assessment of 'no stress' is no longer identical with a favourable prognosis, and notwithstanding the fact that no serious tensions are found the chance of recovery may be small on somatic grounds. This situation was found in a number of patients and will be referred to later on.

'Distress' represents the judgement of the team that the patient is suffering from tensions and conflicts that he is unable to manage; in some cases the bodily illness is closely intertwined with these tensions, and in others the two groups of phenomenon may be distinct. It is, however, judged improbable that the patient will recover as long as the tensions are present, or that he will reach a satisfactory condition even if a somatic recovery is achieved while the distress remains. Therefore, irrespective of the clinical prognosis of the somatic illness, the presence of 'distress' implies that the chance of finding a satisfactory condition on follow-up is smaller than in cases of 'no stress'.

'No stress' thus signifies a favourable prognosis where this is not precluded by the somatic condition, but 'distress' always signifies an unfavourable prognosis.

The prediction of clinical assessment compared to integrated assessment in relation to follow-up.

Table 25 shows that whereas 59 per cent of those judged by the clinical assessment to have a favourable prognosis actually were satisfactory at follow-up, only 31 per cent of those judged to have an unfavourable clinical prognosis had a satisfactory outcome.

Table 25   *Follow-up assessment related to clinical assessment*

follow-up assessment	clinical assessment	
	favourable	unfavourable
condition satisfactory	660 (59%)	157 (31%)
condition unsatisfactory	468 (41%)	345 (70%)
total	1128	502

$\chi^2 = 103.92$ 1 d/f $p < 0.001$ $\gamma = 0.51$

Table 26 shows that whereas 68 per cent of those without distress were satisfactory at follow-up, only 30 per cent of those with distress had a satisfactory outcome. Thus an integrated assessment also helps to predict who will get better.

Table 26   *Follow-up assessment related to team assessment*

follow-up assessment	team assessment		
	no distress	distress	
condition satisfactory	592 (68%)	225 (30%)	817
condition unsatisfactory	279 (32%)	534 (70%)	813
	871	759	1630

$\chi^2 = 237.29$ 1 d/f $p < 0.001$ $\gamma = 0.67$

On the other hand, as is shown in *Table 27*, if we look at the inter-relationship of the three variables (clinical assessment, team assessment, and follow-up assessment) we can then make a much more accurate prediction. Whereas 75 per cent of those with no distress and a favourable

Table 27   *Follow-up assessment related to team and clinical assessments*

	clinical assessment			
	favourable		unfavourable	
	team assessment			
follow-up condition	no distress	distress	no distress	distress
satisfactory	497 (75%)	163 (35%)	95 (46%)	62 (21%)
unsatisfactory	168	300	111	234
total	665	463	206	296 (1630)

$x^2 = 176.03$ 1 d/f $p < 0.001$ $\gamma = 0.69$
$x^2 = 36.85$ 1 d/f $p < 0.001$ $\gamma = 0.53$

clinical prognosis had a satisfactory outcome, only 35 per cent of those with distress and a favourable clinical prognosis did so. A diagrammatic representation of the relationship between the variables is shown in *Figure 8* (see over) from which it can be seen that the presence or absense of distress makes as big a contribution to predicting outcome as the knowledge of the clinical prognosis with which it interacts.

In short, a patient's ability to benefit from a good clinical prognosis depends to a very large effect on the features in his psychological and social background that are indicated by the team's assessment of distress. Patients without 'distress' are more than twice as likely to do well as those considered to be in 'distress'.

Conclusion

This sample of a hospital population brings to mind the warning of Hill (1950): 'It is not too much to say that there is hardly any disease in which a hospital population must not be regarded with suspicion if it is desired to argue from the sample to the universe of all patients.'

There are many reasons for limiting these conclusions to the present sample, but it cannot be denied that something useful may be abstracted from this sample and placed within the frame of reference of more general medical problems. One case of cholera in a hundred-bed hospital will not allow the conclusion that 1 per cent of the general population is

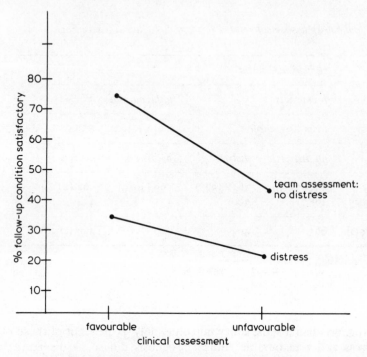

Figure 8   Satisfactory follow-up related to team and clinical assessment

stricken by cholera or even that 1 per cent of all hospital patients is suffering from this disease; but it may be concluded from this one case that the health of the population is seriously threatened. I venture to think that this investigation, independent of the limits of the sample, permits the posing of certain questions concerning the efficiency of the hospital as a link in the chain of aids to health.

It may seem superfluous to demonstrate that the patient who is burdened by cares or conflicts in his private life, will conquer his illness less easily than somebody who is not so burdened. The phenomenon may be self-evident but its consequences remain formidable.

Our investigation has shown that a favourable clinical prognosis was made in 1,128 of 1,630 cases. This means that medical science offered the possibility of recovery to over 69 per cent, but our follow-up showed that only about half (660) of these 1,128 favourable prognoses were realized. Even if the phenomenon of 'distress' is regarded merely as a plodding and worrying attitude to life, or as a psychological peculiarity of the patient, it is plain that such a mental attitude on the part of the patient reduces the efficiency of the hospital by almost half.

This may be self-evident, but it does not have to be accepted as unalterable. Even without following Balint (1957), and postulating that doctor and patient together build the illness, nobody will deny that doctor and patient together bring about recovery. Our investigation has shown that half of the hospital patients to whom the physician may be able to open the way to recovery, are unable to follow him. Perhaps it is true that these people do not recover because they plod along more heavily than others, because their burdens are larger, or their feet less nimble, but in such cases it must be one aspect of therapeutic action to make their going more easy, to lighten the burden, or to smooth their way. The need to give this help (after care, social work, case work, psychotherapy, etc.) must be determined during the stay in hospital, and should be part of the therapeutic programme even if the help to be given is outside the sphere of the hospital itself.

20 Reduction of post-operative pain by encouragement and instruction of patients: a study of doctor–patient rapport

*Lawrence D. Egbert, MD, George E. Battit, MD, Claude E. Welch, MD, & Marshall K. Bartlett, MD**

[*This paper is presented in its original form. The authors are senior anesthetists and surgeons in the USA.*]

Many reports have discussed the treatment of patients suffering after operation. Narcotics are not without danger; they also vary considerably in effectiveness. Hypnosis will reduce pain but is difficult to achieve and requires special training for the operator. Despite considerable effort the problems of treating postoperative pain remain.

Janis has shown that patients who were told about their operations before the procedure remembered the operation and its sequelae more favourably than those who were not well informed. We have determined the effects of instruction, suggestion, and encouragement upon the severity of postoperative pain.

Method

We studied ninety-seven patients after elective intra-abdominal operations (*Table 28* see over). All patients were visited the night before opera-

* extracted from the *New England Journal of Medicine* (1964) **270**: 825–27

tion by the anesthetist, who told them about the preparation for anesthesia, as well as the time and approximate duration of the operation, as warned them that they would wake up in the recovery room. Pre-anesthetic medication, consisting of pentobarbital sodium, 2 mg. per kilogram of body weight, and atropine, 0.6 mg., was administered intramuscularly approximately one hour before operation. Induction of anesthesia was accomplished with thiopental sodium; intubation of the trachea was performed on all patients. Anesthesia was maintained with ether and cyclopropane or nitrous oxide and curare.

The patients were divided into two groups by random order; fifty-one patients (control group) were not told about postoperative pain by the anesthetist. The 'special care' group consisted of forty-six patients who were told about postoperative pain. They were informed where they would feel pain, how severe it would be, and how long it would last and were reassured that having pain was normal after abdominal operations. As soon as the patients appeared aware of the nature of the suffering that would begin on the following day, they were told what would be done about the pain. They were advised that pain is caused by spasm of the muscles under the incision and that they could relieve most of the pain themselves by relaxing these muscles. They could achieve relaxation by slowly taking a deep breath and consciously allowing the abdominal wall to relax. Also, they were shown the use of a trapeze that was hanging over the middle of the bed (control patients also had the trapeze but were not instructed by the anesthetist). Special-care patients were taught how to turn onto one side by using their arms and legs while relaxing their abdominal muscles. Finally, they were told that at first they would find it difficult to relax completely. If they could not achieve a reasonable level of comfort, they should request medication. The presentation was given in a manner of enthusiasm and confidence; the patients were not informed that we were conducting a study. The surgeons, not knowing which patients were receiving special care, continued their practices as usual.

After the operations, narcotics were ordered by the surgical residents; these were later administered by the ward nurses, who were also unaware that we were studying these patients. After the patients were discharged we tabulated the total dose of morphine in milligrams for the first five twenty-four-hour periods after the operation. When meperidine had been administered, we assumed 100 mg. of meperidine to be equal to 10 mg. of morphine (Lasagna and Beecher (1954) indicated that 'meperidine, in parenteral doses of 50 to 100 mg., was at least as good as 10 mg. of morphine in incidence and duration of pain relief'); 60 mg. of codeine was assumed to be nearly equal to 10 mg. of morphine.

During the afternoon after the operation (day zero) the anesthetist visited his patients receiving special care. He reiterated what he had taught the patients the night before and reassured them that the pain they were experiencing was normal; they were again told to request pain medication whenever they could not make themselves tolerably comfortable. The anesthetist listened to their breathing and encouraged them to take a deep breath and relax. All this was repeated on the morning after operation and once or twice a day until they had no further need of narcotics.

On the first and second postoperative days fifty-seven of the patients were visited by an anesthetist whom the patients had not met and who was not aware of the type of treatment being received. This independent observer attempted to record without bias the patients' evaluations about their pain as well as his own impressions from their appearance.

Comparisons of differences between the two groups were made with the use of the t test.

Results

Table 28 shows the types of operations done and the anesthetics given. The average age of the patients in the control group was 52.2 years; in the special-care group the average age of the patients was fifty-two years. There were seventeen men in each group. Randomization in the selection of patients seems to have been satisfactory.

Table 28 *Types of operations and anesthetics**

procedure	control group no. of patients	special-care group no. of patients
operations:		
cholecystectomy	15	17
hiatus hernia	4	1
gastrectomy	9	8
bowel resection	9	6
colectomy	6	9
hysterectomy	6	4
ventral hernia	2	1
Totals	51	46
anesthesia:		
cyclopropane & ether	31	27
nitrous oxide & curare	20	19

* differences not statistically significant

Figure 9 compares the narcotic requirements of the patients. On the day of operation the difference was not statistically significant. For the next five days, however, patients receiving special care requested less narcotics ($p < 0.01$).

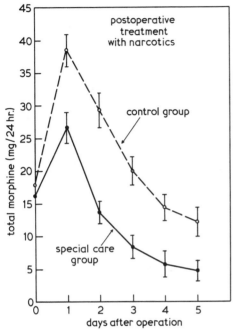

Figure 9   Postoperative treatment with narcotics (means for each day ± standard error of the mean)

All the suggestions given the special-care patients favored a reduction in postoperative narcotics. *Table 29* (see over) shows that these patients did not suffer through the postoperative course just to please the doctor. The independent observer recorded that the special-care patients appeared to be more comfortable and in better physical and emotional condition than the control group. This was emphasized by the surgeons, who, although unaware of the care each patient received, sent the special-care patients home an average of 2.7 days earlier than the control group ($p < 0.01$).

Discussion

Approximately nine out of every ten patients will respond at some time to placebo therapy for postoperative pain; this time of emotional stress is readily modified by psychotherapy. Placebo effect may be defined as

Table 29 *Pains on the first and second days after operation (averages ± standard errors)*

postoperative day	severity of pain*	
	control group (30 patients)	special-care group (27 patients)
1st:		
subjective report	1.768 ± 0.200	1.591 ± 0.205
objective report	1.735 ± 0.191	1.187 ± 0.192†
2nd:		
subjective report	1.333 ± 0.188	0.966 ± 0.195
objective report	1.333 ± 0.216	0.827 ± 0.172‡

* pain graded as follows: severe, + + +, moderate, + +, mild, +, and almost none, o
† difference statistically significant ($p < 0.05$)
‡ approaches significance ($p < 0.1$)

one that is not attributable to a specific pharmacologic property of the treatment; the effects of placebos are readily modified by suggestion and depend upon the symbolic implications of the physician and his ministrations. We believe that our discussions with patients have changed the meaning of the postoperative situation for these patients. By utilizing an active placebo action, we have been able to reduce their postoperative pain.

Others have shown that talking out anxieties and understanding the source of anxiety helps patients. Our data demonstrate that anesthetists, untrained in hypnotism or formal psychiatry, may nevertheless have a very powerful effect on their patients. We have previously shown that this reassurance (we call it 'superficial psychotherapy') can be started during the preoperative visit; it should be continued into the postoperative period.

It should be pointed out that a great deal more work is involved in this practice of anesthesia than in the customary practice of anesthesia. We found that our methods of talking to patients changed during the study – for example, one of our early patients became hysterical during the discussion about postoperative pain; and we now know it is wise to build up the discussion slowly in patients who become too frightened. Nevertheless, retreating from the frightened patient before operation exposes that patient to greater psychic stress during the postoperative period. The patient who persistently avoids discussing these problems before he is operated on is a particularly troublesome patient later. Another error was of interest: one patient was seen before operation and anesthetized, and then the anesthetist went on vacation without notifying the patient or surgeon. Upon seeing the patient five days later, the anesthetist was greeted with great annoyance ('Where the hell have you been?') by the patient. To balance these errors, we found that almost none of the patients in the special care group had the complaint, 'Why didn't you tell me it was going to be like this?' – which was not uncommon in the control group. Each patient has his own personal psychologic makeup; each patient needs 'special' treatment, tailored to meet his own particular psychologic needs.

The specialty of anesthesia has been criticized sharply as lacking in involvement with patient care and responsibility. Our data show that an anesthetist is able to establish rapport with surgical patients and that a useful purpose is served by this contact. Since the sole purpose of the anesthetist in administering anesthesia is to reduce pain associated with operations, it appears reasonable for him to consider the whole job. The anesthetist who understands his patient and who believes that each patient is 'his' patient ceases to be merely a clever technician in the operating room.

The effect of encouragement and education on ninety-seven surgical patients was studied. 'Special-care' patients were told what to expect during the postoperative period; they were then taught how to relax, how to take deep breaths, and how to move so that they would remain more comfortable after operation. Comparing these patients with a control group of patients, we were able to reduce the postoperative narcotic requirements by half. Patients who were encouraged during the immediate postoperative period by their anesthetists were considered by their surgeons ready for discharge from the hospital 2.7 days before the control patients. We believe that if an anesthetist considers himself a doctor who alleviates pain associated with operations, he must realize that only part of his work is in the operating rooms; the patients need ward care by their anesthetists as well.

21 Children, stress, and hospitalization: a field experiment

James K. Skipper, Jr & Robert C. Leonard*

[*The lengthy original of this paper is carefully and tightly argued. In addition to providing detailed data on the experiments' effects on blood pressure, pulse rate, and post-operative emesis, the authors also did this for temperature, fluid intake, nurses' assessment of adaptation to hospital, the mothers' post-admission telephone calls to the hospital, fever, and the children's fears, crying, and disturbed sleep. In this version these results have been reported without the convincing supporting tables. Otherwise the paper was edited according to the editors' general strategy. The authors are sociologists now working at the Virginia Polytechnic Institute and State University (USA) and the University of Arizona (USA), respectively.*]

This paper reports an experimental study concerned with the reduction of some of the effects of hospitalization and surgery – physiological as well as social and psychological – in young children. Usually much of children's behavior while hospitalized for surgery is presumed to be a response to psychological and physiological stress. This research offers evidence demonstrating the effects of *social interaction* on children's response to hospitalization for a tonsillectomy operation.

The data in this report are based on a field experiment designed to test the effects on the behavior of hospitalized children of nurses' interaction with the children's mothers. We postulate that hospitalization for a tonsillectomy operation is likely to produce a great deal of stress for child patients and their mothers. For the children this stress is likely to result in: elevated temperature, pulse rate, and blood pressure; disturbed sleep; postoperative vomiting; a delayed recovery period; and other forms of behavior which deviate from the medical culture's

*extracted from the *Journal of Health and Social Behavior* (1968) 9: (4) 275–87, December

norms of 'health' and normal progress of hospitalization and treatment.

We conceptualize these patient behaviors to be simply instances of individual human behavior, which therefore can be affected by the patient's attitudes, feelings, and beliefs about his medical treatment, hospital care, and those who provide it. This is not to disregard physical and physiological variables as stimuli for the patient's response, or to deny that the response may be 'physiological'. Rather, we reason that in addition the meaning the patient attaches to the stimuli will also affect his response.

Past attempts at reducing children's stress in the hospital have not fully considered the effect that parents and especially the mother may have on the child's level of emotional tension (Prugh et al. 1953). If the mother were able to manage her own stress and be calm, confident, and relaxed, this might be communicated to the child and ease his distress. Moreover, the mother might be more capable of making rational decisions concerning her child's needs and thus facilitate his adaptation to the hospital situation. An important means of reducing stress from potentially threatening events is through the communication of information about the event (Janis 1958). This allows the individual to organize his thoughts, actions, and feelings about the event. It provides a framework to appraise the potentially frightening and disturbing perceptions which one might actually experience. An individual is able to engage in an imaginative mental rehearsal in which the 'work of worrying' can take place. According to Janis (1958) the information is likely to be most effective if communicated in the context of interest, support, and reassurance on the part of authoritative individuals.

Regular and experimental conditions

We can describe the usual routine staff approach to tonsillectomy patients and their mothers from the experience of members of our research team who worked for several months in advance of the study on the ward where our experiments were conducted. Typically, the staff approached the patient as a work object on which to perform a set of tasks, rather than as a participant in the work process or an individual who needs help in adjusting to a new environment. The attending surgeon's interaction with the child was limited primarily to the performance of the operation and release from the hospital. The nursing staff tended to initiate interaction only when they needed some data for their charts or had to perform an instrumental act such as taking blood pressure, checking fluid intake, or giving a medication. The typical role was the bureaucratic one of information gatherer, chart assembler, and order deliverer. They offered very little information and were usually evasive if questioned directly. If the mother displayed stress, the staff tried to ignore it or to get her to leave the ward.

For our research purposes, actual practice made a good comparison condition against which to test the hypothesis that: the children's stress can be reduced indirectly by reducing the stress of the mothers. The experimental approach began with the admission of the mother and child to the hospital. Although the child was present, the focus of inter-action was the mother. No more attention was paid to the child than under routine (control) admission conditions. The special nurse attempted to create an atmosphere which would facilitate the communication of information to the mother, maximize freedom to verbalize her fear, anxiety, and special problems, and to ask any and all questions which were on her mind. The information given to the mother tried to paint an accurate picture of the reality of the situation. Mothers were told what routine events to expect and when they were likely to occur – including the actual time schedule for the operation.

The special nurse probed the mother's feelings and the background of those feelings as possible causes of stress regardless of what the topic might be, or where it might lead. In each individual case the special nurse tried to help the mother meet her own individual problems.

With the experimental group, the process of admission took an average of about five minutes longer than regular admission procedures. In addition to the interaction which took place at admission, the special nurse met with the mothers of the first twenty-four experimental group patients for about five minutes at several other times when potentially stressful events were taking place. These times were: 6.00 and 8.00 p.m. the evening of the operation; and at discharge the following day. The remaining sixteen experimental group mothers were seen only at admission. For purposes of analysis the first twenty-four patients and their controls constitute experiment I, and the remaining sixteen patients and their controls experiment II.

Our theory predicts that: providing the experimental communication for the mothers of children hospitalized for tonsillectomy would result in less stress, a change in the mothers' definition of the situation, and different behavioral responses. This in turn would result in less stress for the child and, hopefully, a 'better' adaptation to the hospitalization and surgery. If this could be demonstrated, not only might it be a practical means of reducing the stress of young children hospitalized for tonsillectomy, but it would also provide direct evidence on the effect of social interaction on behaviors often assumed to be responses to psychological stress.

Research methodology

To test these hypotheses an experiment was conducted at one large teaching hospital, in a four-month period during the late fall and winter. The sample included all patients between the ages of three and nine years admitted to the hospital for tonsillectomy and having no previous hospital experience. Patients were excluded from the sample if there were known complicating medical conditions, their parents did not speak English, or their mothers did not accompany them through admission procedures. A total of eighty patients qualified for the sample. Forty-eight of the children were male, and thirty-two were female. Thirty-six were between the ages of three and five, and forty-four between the ages of six and nine. Thirty-three of the mothers had more than twelve years of formal education, forty-five between ten and twelve years, and two less than ten years. All the families were able to pay for the cost of the operation and the hospitalization.

Children were admitted to the hospital late in the afternoon the day before surgery was performed. At admission each child received a physical examination which included securing samples of blood and urine and a check on weight, blood pressure, temperature, and pulse rate. When the admission procedures were completed the child was dressed in his night clothes and taken to one of two four-bed rooms limited to children who were to undergo a tonsillectomy. Control and experimental patients were not separated, but placed in rooms with each other to eliminate any systematic peer influence. From midnight until their return to the room after surgery, the children were not allowed to take fluids. The next morning, starting at eight o'clock, the children were taken to the operating room, one every half-hour. Each child voided before the surgery. Following the operation they were taken to the recovery room where they remained until awake. Then they were returned to their room where they stayed until their discharge late the following morning. Only six of the mothers gained permission to 'room in' with their child overnight. Three of these were in the control group and three were in the experimental group. All but one of the remaining mothers was able to spend most of the operation day at the hospital. However, a record was not kept of the actual amount of time spent with her child. In fact it was beyond the resources of this investigation to obtain systematic data on the mother–child interaction; that is, the actual differences in frequency, timing, and quality of interaction between control and experimental group mothers with their children.

The study was experimental in the sense that R. A. Fisher's (1947) classic design was used. The children were randomly assigned to control and experimental groups. No significant differences were found in the composition of the groups on the basis of: sex, age, or health of the children, age of the mothers, class background, religious affiliation, and types of anesthesia used during the operation. Since the children were randomly assigned, antecedent variations and their consequences are taken into account by the probability test.

Correlated measurement bias may be a much more important source of mistaken conclusion than bias in the composition of the groups. One way of gaining some control of this type of bias is a 'blind' procedure in which the individual measuring the dependent variables does not know which treatment the subjects have been assigned. With one exception, blind procedures were employed in this research.

The independent variable in the experiment was interaction. The experimental manipulations were all communicative – affective as well as cognitive. They emphasized the communication of information and emotional support to the mothers. The dependent variable was the behavior of the children. Thus the experimental variation was the interaction under usual hospital conditions compared with what was added experimentally.

All patients and their mothers whether in control or experimental groups were subjected to regular hospital treatment and procedures. In addition, experimental group patients and mothers were admitted to the hospital by a specially trained nurse. Admission is a crucial time to introduce the experimental communication. Entry into any new social situation can be a tense experience. Lack of attention to the patient's definition of the situation in the admission process not only does not relieve stress but may actually increase it. Previous experimentation (Leonard, Skipper, and Woolridge 1967) has indicated the potential effect of providing such attention on immediate stress and also the patient's adjustment to the hospital experience.

The regular nursing staff was informed that a study was in progress and asked to complete a short questionnaire regarding the behavior of the child and mother, as well as making charts and records available. They did not know which patients were in the control and experimental groups. The study was conducted at a teaching hospital, and the staff was used to having all sorts of projects taking place on the ward. They had become immune to them and ignored them unless they seriously interfered with their work. The staff was also familiar with the research personnel, who had been working on various projects on the ward on and off for over a year.

At admission, regardless of group, each mother was asked if she would be willing to complete a short questionnaire which would be mailed to her eight days after her child was discharged, and would concern the hospital experience and its aftermath. None of the mothers refused. The mothers were not aware of whether they were in the control or experimental group. The questionnaire asked for the mother's perception of: her own level of stress before, during, and after the operation, as well as her possible distress about a future similar operation; her desire for information during the hospitalization and her feeling of helpfulness; her trust and confidence in the medical and nursing staff; and her general satisfaction with the hospital experience. By means of a second questionnaire administered to the regular nursing staff, an independent measure of each mother's level of stress and general adaptation to the hospital experience was secured. To discover the effects of hospitalization on the child after discharge, a section of the mailback questionnaire to the mother also concerned aspects of the child's behavior during his first seven days at home. Items were related to such matters as whether it was necessary to call a physician, and whether the child recovered during the first week at home. In addition, mothers were asked if their child manifested any unusual behavior which might be regarded as an emotional reaction to the operation and hospitalization such as disturbed sleep, vomiting, finicky eating, crying, fear of doctors and nurses, etc.

Based on previous research several somatic measures of children's stress in the hospital were selected. Each child's temperature, systolic blood pressure, and pulse rate were recorded at four periods during the hospitalization: admission, preoperatively, postoperatively, and at discharge. The normal variability of these vital signs is not great in children between the ages of three and nine. Children at this age have not developed effective inhibiting mechanisms, so that an increase in excitement, apprehension, anxiety, fear, etc. will be reflected in the level of these indicators. Inability to void postoperatively and postoperative emesis also may be responses to stress over which a child has little conscious control. The time of first voiding after the operation was recorded as well as the incidence of emesis from the time the child entered the recovery room until discharge. Finally, the amount of fluids a child is able to consume after the operation may be related to the mother's understanding of its importance and her ability to get the child to cooperate. Fluid intake was recorded for the first seven hours upon the child's return from the recovery room. This period represented the shortest time that any mother in the study stayed with her child after the operation.

Systolic blood pressure was measured and recorded by the special nurse. Checks on the objectivity and reliability of the special nurse were made periodically. Data on pulse rate, temperature, postoperative vomiting, ability to void postoperatively, and oral intake of fluids were collected and recorded by staff nurses who had no knowledge of which children had been assigned to the control and experimental groups.

Data were complete on all patients and mothers with two exceptions. First, since reliability checks were not made on the special nurses' measurement of systolic blood pressure for several patients in experiment II, these were not used. Second, the regular nursing staff's estimate of the mothers' stress and adaptation was not available for two mothers in experiment II. The response rate to the mailback questionnaire was over 92 per cent, seventy-four of the eighty mothers returning the questionnaire. Four of the nonreturns were control group mothers (two in experiment I and two in experiment II) and two experimental group mothers (experiment I). All hypotheses predicted the direction of differences between control group mothers and experimental group mothers and children.

Findings

In a previous paper (Skipper, Leonard, and Rhymes 1968) the effect of the special nurse's interaction with the mothers was presented in detail. In summary, according to the mothers' reports on the mail-back

Table 30 *Mean systolic blood pressure of control and experimental children at four periods during hospitalization*

	admission	preoperative 8.00 p.m.		postoperative 8.00 p.m.		discharge		total N
	$\bar{x}$	$\bar{x}$	t^*	$\bar{x}$	t^*	$\bar{x}$	t^*	
experiment I								
experimental	111.5	109.1	4.81 $P < .0005$	109.7	7.73 $P < .0005$	104.7	6.81 $P < .0005$	24
control	110.4	120.3		127.8		120.9		24

* one tailed test

questionnaire, experimental group mothers suffered less stress than control group mothers during and after the operation. This finding was substantiated by the independent evaluation of the regular nursing staff. The regular nursing staff also estimated each mother's difficulty in adapting to the hospitalization. Experimental group mothers were rated as having less over-all difficulty in adaptation. This agreed with the mother's own self-evaluation. Experimental group mothers, as compared to control group mothers, reported: less lack of information during the hospitalization, less difficulty in feeling helpful to their child, and a greater degree of satisfaction with the total hospital experience. Taken together these measures provide evidence in support of the hypothesis that social interaction with the special nurse was an effective means of changing the mothers' definition of the situation to lower stress levels, thus allowing them to make a more successful adaptation to the hospitalization and operation.

In this paper we are concerned with the effect of the nurse-mother interaction on the children.

At admission, the differences in systolic blood pressure were, of course, random, with the experimental mean actually slightly higher than the control (*Table 30*). This difference was reversed after the experimental treatment, and the control children continued to have higher average blood pressure throughout their hospital stay. In experiment I the mean for experimental group children at admission, 111.5, dropped preoperatively to 109.1, remained relatively the same postoperatively, 109.7, and then dropped sharply at discharge to 104.7. The discharge mean was lower than the admission mean. The mean for control group children at admission, 110.4, rose to 120.3 preoperatively, and continued to rise to 127.8 postoperatively, before falling to 120.9 at discharge. The discharge mean was much higher than the admission mean. The mean differences between the control and experimental group children reached a level of statistical significance of beyond .005,

Table 31 *Mean pulse rate of control and experimental children at four periods during hospitalization*

	admission	preoperative 8.00 p.m.		postoperative 8.00 p.m.		discharge		total N
	$\bar{x}$	$\bar{x}$	t^*	$\bar{x}$	t^*	$\bar{x}$	t^*	
experiment I								
experimental	103.6	95.8	5.10	101.6	6.31	95.2	5.08	24
			$P<.0005$		$P<.0005$		$P<.0005$	
control	104.6	110.8		122.2		110.8		24
experiment II								
experimental	105.6	100.2	1.38	117.1	.83	105.4	2.13	16
			$P<.10$		$P>.10$		$P<.025$	
control	104.9	107.5		123.1		116.8		16

* one tailed test

preoperatively, postoperatively, and at discharge. As mentioned previously, the data for experiment II are not presented since reliability checks on the special nurses' measurement of systolic blood pressure were not available for several patients. However, the data that were available followed the same patterns as described in experiment I.

We see in *Table 31* (see back) that in both experiments there was little difference at admission between the mean pulse rate of control and experimental group children. In experiment I the mean for experimental group children at admission, 103.6, dropped to 95.8 preoperatively, rose to 101.6 postoperatively, and then fell to 95.2 at discharge. The discharge mean was lower than the admission mean. The control group mean at admission, 104.6, rose preoperatively to 110.8 and continued to rise to 122.2 postoperatively, before falling only to 110.8 at discharge. The discharge mean in the control set was much greater than the admission mean. The mean difference between the two groups reached a statistical level of significance beyond .005 at each of the periods. Exactly the same pattern appeared in experiment II, but the differences between the group means were considerably less and did not reach a high level of statistical significance.

Further data shows that in both experiments I and II at admission there was little difference between the mean temperature of control and experimental children. In experiment I the experimental group mean at admission, 99.4, fell to 99.1 preoperatively, rose to 100.1 postoperatively and dropped to 99.2 at discharge. Again, as in the case of systolic blood pressure and pulse rate, the discharge mean was lower than the admission mean. The control group mean at admission, 99.5, rose to 99.8 preoperatively and continued to rise to 100.7 postoperatively before falling to 99.8 at discharge. Again the mean discharge figure for the control group children was higher than the admission mean. The same pattern appeared in experiment II.

In addition to systolic blood pressure, pulse rate, and temperature, the children's postoperative emesis, hour of first voiding, and oral intake of fluids were checked. *Table 32* shows that in experiment I, ten of the children vomited after the operation, seven of them more than once, while only three experimental group children vomited, none of them more than once. Although the incidence of postoperative emesis was not as great in experiment II as experiment I, the same pattern appeared. Control group children experienced more emesis than experimental group children. Furthermore, control group children did not void as rapidly after the operation as experimental group children. In experiment I the mean hour of first voiding for control group children was well over seven and one-half hours compared to four and one-half hours for experimental group children. In experiment II the corresponding figures were; control group children approximately six and three-quarter hours and experimental group children five and three-quarter hours.

Table 32   *Incidence of postoperative emesis for control and experimental children*

| | postoperative emesis | | | | | | | |
| | none | | once | | more than once | | | |
	N	%	N	%	N	%	total N	x^2
experiment I								
control	14	58	3	12	7	29	24	$x^2 = 8.40$
experimental	21	88	3	12	0	0	24	$P < .01$
total	35	73	6	12	7	15	48	
experiment II								
control	12	75	1	6	3	19	16	$x^2 = 1.15$
experimental	14	88	1	6	1	6	16	$P < .10$
total	26	81	2	6	4	12	32	

Moreover, in both experiments control children consumed much less fluid during the first seven hours after the operation than experimental group children.

Taken together, these physiological measures indicate that the level of stress among experimental children was much lower. This was true for both experiments. Experimental children had lower mean levels of systolic blood pressure, pulse rate, and temperature preoperatively, postoperatively, and at discharge than control group children. Experimental group children had less postoperative emesis, voided earlier, and drank more fluids than control group children. These data lend support to the hypothesis that the experimental nurse-mother interaction would reduce mothers' stress and increase their ability to adapt rationally to the hospitalization, which, in turn, would have profound effects on their children. The hypothesis is further supported by the regular nursing staffs' evaluation of the children's general over-all adaptation to the hospitalization. By means of a short questionnaire each staff nurse who had the most contact with a child was asked to judge whether she considered the child's adaptation to be high, average, or low. The staff nurses had no knowledge of whether a child was in the control or experimental group. In experiment I 50 per cent of the experimental group children were judged as making a high adaptation to the hospitalization compared to only 17 per cent of control group children. The corresponding figures for experiment II were: experimental group children 56 per cent high adaptation and control group children 31 per cent high adaptation.

The mail-back questionnaire to the mothers provides data on the children's condition and behavior at home during the first week after discharge. These data indicate the experimental group children seemed to experience, physiologically, less ill effects from the operation and hospitalization and made a more rapid recovery than control group children. In addition, major differences were found in three areas: excessive crying, disturbed sleep, and an unusual fear of doctors, nurses, and hospitals.

PART VII
The organization of hospitals

PART SIX
The Grammar of Inheritance

22 The sociology of time and space in an obstetrical hospital

William R. Rosengren & Spencer DeVault*

[*This paper has been reduced from the original by only a small amount in accordance with the editors' general strategy. The authors are Professors of Sociology in the USA.*]

The observations that formed the basis for this essay were made in a large lying-in hospital in the United States. In a four-month period we spent some 150 hours observing in this delivery service. This was done in connection with two independent studies of social psychological factors in pregnancy. Our procedures were simple. On the days (or nights) on which we came to the hospital, we were provided with a room in the residents' quarters, and supplied with hospital uniforms, caps, masks, and insulated shoes. We then observed all the activities of the service, talked informally with the staff during coffee breaks, while relaxing in the lounges, and in the work situations.

All our observations were independently recorded when time permitted, with both of us working from a general outline of factors for which to search. We both recorded the typical fieldnote type of material, and we compared them after each observational experience. Our original

* extracted from chapter 9, in Eliot Friedson (ed.), *The Hospital in Modern Society* (1964) New York: The Free Press: 266–91

purpose was not that of posing questions about the social organization of the delivery service. As time went on, however, we were increasingly impressed that the behavior of the personnel seemed to differ markedly, depending upon where it took place and in what sequence.

Following these initial leads, we found it useful to consider our experiences under these general rubrics:

1 The *spatial* distribution of activities in the delivery service in so far as certain regions appeared to be set aside for particular modes of behaviour and attitudes – staff to staff, and staff to patients. That is, it became increasingly clear that both attitudes and overt behavior of the several functionaries in the service – patients, nurses, and doctors – varied, depending upon the particular place in which they might be found.

2 The *segregation* of behaviors, one from the other, in so far as persons occupying the same status appeared to behave differently in different places, depending upon the ecological factors involved in each place – its position in temporal sequences, its physical symbols, and the ways in which each place was physically separated from other places. In other words, the differences in behavior that were noted to be dependent upon particular areas were not fully a function of purposive choice on the part of either the personnel or the patients, but they were both sanctioned by the normative system and elicited by the nature of the physical settings themselves.

3 The *rhythm* of activities – the periodicity with which events took place to the extent that the behavior of the personnel was organized and patterned in terms of regularities of occurrence.

4 The *tempo* of activities – the number of events, both social and physiological, that occurred within any given unit of time. Important here is the fact that the temporal organization of the hospital was, in part, a function of the continual imperfection balance between the physiological and functional organization of activities.

5 The *timing* of activities – the coordination of separate and diverse pulsations – both physiological and functional – in so far as different rhythms and tempos were taking place at the same time. It was by means of timing sequences, therefore, that temporal organization could actually take place.

Distribution and segregation of activities: barriers and atmospheres

The obstetrical service is schematically represented in *Figure 10*. Each region in the service is itself set apart in several ways from the others. This segregation appears to be accomplished not only by space but also by rules of dress, of expected behavior, and of decorum – all of which serve to indicate the dissimilarity of each place, as well as to present an image of the place that might cast both patients and staff into desired roles with respect to one another.

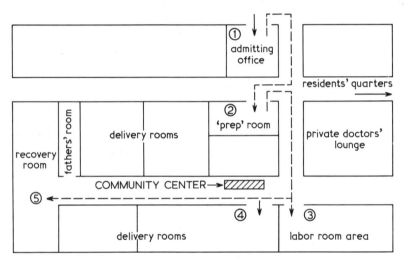

Figure 10   Map of the obstetrical service. Arrows indicate route taken by patients.

The admitting office is just beyond the residents' quarters. Significantly, perhaps, here there are no barriers of any kind – not even doors – almost as a symbol of welcome to the incoming patient. A mood of friendly casualness characterizes the behavior of the admitting room staff, and it is here where the staff is most casual in regard to decorum in both attitudes and dress. This is consistent with the function of the admitting office as the intermediary stage in the hospitalization of the patient, for the physical setting, its spatial location, and the behavior of personnel in it serve as a gradual introduction of the patient to the new world of the service.

Directly opposite the admitting room is the preparation or 'prep' room where the incoming patient is stripped of her self-image as 'person', and cast most effectively and promptly into her new status of 'medical phenomenon'. Of interest to us as observers, we were invited into the prep room only when it was occupied by an unmarried, lower-class Negro prostitute. Until that time we were told almost nothing of what took place in 'prepping', nor were we told the names of those who worked there or their occupational status. Segregation of the prep room was accomplished not only by physical and symbolic barriers but also by an atmosphere of anonymity exceeded nowhere else in the service.

In the area of the labor rooms, one is isolated from the nurses in charge, and from the patients, by a sturdy shoulder-high and seemingly non-functional barricade. This not only segregates the patients from those who pass by but also symbolically segregates the attending nurses from others in the hospital. Perhaps implicit in this mode of segregation is the notion that the nurses are definitely 'in charge' and that others in service have no authority beyond that point. Also, the physical barrier – serving to maintain status differences – seemed to us to be reinforced symbolically by the dim lighting and drab decor of the interior of the labor rooms. The staff was in agreement that the patients seemed to 'behave better' while in labor under the quieting effect of the gray decor of the rooms. At the same time, here the nurse was most likely to conduct herself with most confidence in the role of the nurse in the presence of other personnel, and perhaps least like a nurse when interacting only with other nurses. From a slightly different perspective, both the physical and the symbolic segregation of the labor rooms may be understood to be a function of labor as a kind of 'deviant' activity in the service. That is, there is none of the 'highlighting' of the place or of the patients here to suggest that what takes place in the region is actually germane to the entire process.

Thus far we have discussed some of the regions of the service in terms of spatial and segregational aspects as if they had distinct boundaries. Of course, this is not true; if it were, it would suggest that moods, attitudes, and behaviors had discrete boundaries as well. It is more proper to speak of the overlapping of regional boundaries – a frame of reference that may account for the periodic times and occasional places where the behavior patterns among the staff are less clear and distinct than they are when one is observing well within a bounded area.

The administrative nurses hold forth in the area of the delivery rooms. At this point – which is really the 'community center' and the point of both physiological and social climax – we found it interesting to note that the projected image of the hospital and consequently, the expected roles and attitudes of both staff and patient are cast most effectively by symbols – uniforms, stainless steel, medicines with their odors, brilliant lighting, and so forth.

The operating arena is just beyond the delivery room; it is segregated from the rest of the service by a wide red line painted wall to wall and ceiling to floor. No one without surgical cap, face mask, and insulated shoes is allowed beyond that point. During our first conducted tour of the service we entered that region without the required accoutrements – perhaps because we were not yet really considered a 'part' of the scene.

Further along this corridor, and perhaps significantly furthest from the community center, is the recovery room. This is a large, dimly-lit room attended by one nurse. The functions here are also of the 'deviant' variety. The mother is relegated here after delivery of the child, while the newborn is retained in the community center where much attention is paid to it by high-status personnel – obstetricians and pediatricians. This spatial indication of the importance of the child is reinforced by timing sequences, and the value placed on the child may, in fact, account for the emphasis that is placed upon administering anesthesia. Without anesthesia the patient may become troublesome to the obstetric team, and their reassuring and comforting gestures towards the patient often give way to irritability.

The 'fathers' room' is adjacent to the recovery room – unattended and suggestive that the father is regarded as the least important person in the process. By its sparseness of furnishing, its physical isolation, and its small size, this room seemed to communicate symbolically the idea that the fathers are unnecessary and functionally peripheral.

In terms of spatial patterns, it would appear that the extent of spatial segregation relates to the value placed upon the activities in the region relative to the 'business' or 'goals' of the establishment. That is, those areas that are most dispensable with regard to the delivery of babies are those that are spatially most apart from the community center. Physical segregation, on the other hand, seemed to be most related to status differences among the staff members – doors, walls, counters, and the like. Finally, symbolic forms of segregation between regions appeared to us to be most related to the communication of organizationally appropriate attitudes and values – colors, odors, lighting, signs, and so forth. Whereas physical segregation served in some sense to declare gradations in status, symbolic forms of segregation appeared more to articulate roles.

A substantive example: the ecology of pain

To express more fully the interrelationships between time, space, and social behavior, we turn now to a specific substantive area: the ways in which the hospital is organized to define, legitimatize, sanction, and handle the expression of pain by patients.

There are, first of all, certain places in the service where pain is legitimatized and defined as such, and others in which it is not. By and large, pain is not sanctioned in any place other than the delivery room, for it is only here that the hospital provides the means to handle pain in an affectively neutral fashion – namely, anesthesia. The acceptance or sanctioning of pain in any other region – the admitting room, the prep room, and even the labor rooms – would necessitate a more personalized orientation towards the patient by the staff, rather than by the technical, mechanical, and personally neutral means that are so characteristic of the delivery room. This is not to say that women are in pain only in the delivery room, but merely that it is neither accepted nor dealt with as such by the staff – particularly high-status staff. And not only does the staff segregate pain in this spatial sense, but this meaning appears to be shared by the patients as well – many patients seem a bit apologetic about having pain when in these other regions. In places not sanctioning pain, when the patient's discomfort intrudes itself upon the staff, various means are employed to cope with it in an affectively neutral fashion. In the prep room it is handled by the use of humor and comparatively low-status personnel; in the labor room, not only by the more intimate contact taking place between patient and low-status personnel but also by defining the phenomenon as something other than pain – complaining, pampering, nervousness, or what have you; and in the recovery room by its spatial and symbolic segregation as well as by defining it as unconscious behavior of one who is still under the effects of anesthesia.

The symbolism of lighting, individual segregation of patients, and perhaps even the mood and attitudes of the nurses on duty, serve to minimize the patient's attempts to legitimatize her discomfort as genuine pain. Spatially there appeared to be a kind of gradient as to the legitimation of pain, with the greater sanctioning of pain found the closer the 'place' was to the delivery rooms, and a corresponding decrease as one moved away from the community center. Significantly, it is in this 'climax' region of the delivery room, where pain is most fully sanctioned and accepted by the staff, that the affectively neutral orientation is most likely to break down. For here – perhaps for the first time – the entire obstetrical team is confronted, and at close quarters, with the patient and her discomfort. She is highlighted not only in a physical and inter-actional sense but in an organizational sense as well. An important relation between status and 'place' is clearly evident here because the anesthetist has no part to play in the labor room, even though the manifestation of pain there may actually be as great as, or even greater than, that shown in the delivery room. Once pain is accepted as such – in the delivery room – there is then a special functionary to handle it in an affectively neutral fashion: the anesthetist. Pain is not only sanctioned in the delivery room; it is expected, too. If there is no pain, this would mean that the anesthetist, who occupies a position of con-siderable prestige, would be superfluous. Moreover, the legitimation of pain is also organized temporally. There are patterns according to which pain is sanctioned and expected – only so often and for only so long. To show pain either too frequently or too infrequently or, indeed, not at all, is disrupting to the obstetrical team.

23 Institutionalism and schizophrenia: summary, discussion, and conclusions

John K. Wing & George W. Brown*

[*This reading is taken from the final chapter of a book describing a long and carefully designed enquiry into the influence of the hospital environment on schizophrenic patients. The measures of the ward environment, of patient attitudes, of the patient's condition, etc, are all described in earlier chapters and were done carefully and after much work along the lines of those measures discussed in Readings 1, 2, and 8 of this volume. The authors are Professor of Social Psychiatry and of Sociology respectively, in the UK.*]

The various stages of this study point towards a conclusion which is very difficult to resist – that a substantial proportion, though by no means all, of the morbidity shown by long-stay schizophrenic patients in mental hospitals is a product of their environment. The social pressures which act to produce this extra morbidity can to some extent be counteracted, but the process of reform may itself have a natural history and an end. We should like now to discuss these propositions in detail, both in their theoretical and their practical aspects.

Interaction between clinical and social factors

Poverty of the social environment as a cause of clinical deterioration

The most important hypothesis under test is that certain aspects of the social environment actually cause clinical improvement or deterioration.

* extracted from J. K. Wing, and G. W. Brown, *Institutionalism and Schizophrenia* (1970) Cambridge: Cambridge University Press: 177–94

The first step was to show that, looked at from the patient's point of view, there was a certain uniformity in level of social stimulation. Those who had fewest personal possessions tended to be occupied in the least interesting activities, to be regarded most pessimistically by nurses, to be least in touch with the world outside through letters or visits from relatives or weekends at home, and to spend most time doing absolutely nothing. Conversely, those who were best off according to one index, tended also to be well off according to the others. There was a wide range of social experience in each of the hospitals, but in 1960, Severalls's patients were likely to be most deprived. (Even there, however, one ward had previously been set aside for private patients and the atmosphere was still not unlike that of a genteel boarding house.)

Environmental poverty, measured in these terms, was very highly correlated with a 'clinical poverty syndrome', independently measured, and compounded of social withdrawal, flatness of affect, and poverty of speech. Both environmental and clinical poverty became more intense with length of stay, although they remained highly interrelated when length of stay was allowed for.

The second step was to show that, although the association between clinical and social poverty remained strong in three different mental hospitals, the one with the richest social environment (Netherne) contained patients with the fewest negative symptoms. Even when twenty patients in each hospital were selected because they were equivalent in clinical grouping, degree of social withdrawal, age, length of stay, and attitude to discharge, most of the environmental indices still showed Severalls at a disadvantage.

If the negative symptoms do indeed reflect a fundamental process in schizophrenia and have an important biological component (as suggested in chapter 1, Wing and Brown 1970), it might well be assumed that the direction of cause and effect is from patient to environment; that schizophrenia inevitably creates its own social community. To some extent, this must be so if the staff allows it. Thus, if more severely-ill patients had been admitted to Severalls, they might have given rise to at least part of the difference in social environments. We could not demonstrate that schizophrenic patients admitted to Severalls were any more severely ill than those admitted to Netherne or Mapperley; in fact, the discharge rates of the latter two hospitals were higher, which would work in the opposite direction. Nevertheless, the argument is not conclusive.

Even supposing, however, that the poorer results at Severalls in 1960 were really due to more severely-ill patients being originally admitted there, a test of the social hypothesis is still possible.

If schizophrenic patients are 'vulnerable' to under-stimulating social environments (this being one of their most characteristic impairments), they will react by increased withdrawal even to an environment they have created themselves. An attempt can then be made to reverse the process by appropriate staff action. If the social milieu does improve measurably, there should be a corresponding decrease in 'clinical poverty'. This should be true, not only at Severalls, but at the other hospitals as well.

We had every reason to suppose that, at least at Severalls, considerable efforts would be made to improve the social environment. Further surveys were therefore undertaken which showed that poverty of the social milieu had decreased, at all three hospitals, by 1964, and that the clinical condition of the patients had improved concomitantly. Even more significantly, there was a clear difference between patients whose social surroundings became socially richer, who tended to show fewer negative symptoms, and those whose social environment remained impoverished, who tended not to improve. Changes in drug treatment could not explain these facts.

It is still possible to think of an alternative non-social hypothesis for these results. There is a long-established clinical theory that the schizophrenic process gradually 'burns out'. It could therefore be argued that some patients eventually show improvement whatever their social environment. If so, they would be easier to resocialize, they could more easily be provided with clothes and other equipment, their contacts with the outside world would be easier to increase, and the nurses' attitudes would naturally become more favourable. Hospitals where value is attached to making the social environment more stimulating would take advantage of such opportunities, but the social changes would be a *result*, and not a *cause*, of the clinical improvement.

The major difficulty about accepting this explanation as it stands is that the clinical poverty syndrome was most marked in 1960, when patients had been in hospital, on average, sixteen years, and should have had plenty of time to improve if they were going to do so. However, there is a way of putting both hypotheses to the test since, if the social environment should, for any reason, become socially *more* impoverished, the predictions are quite different. On the burning-out hypothesis, clinical improvement will continue anyway, since it is not dependent on the social milieu. On the social hypothesis, there should be clinical deterioration.

We showed that there was indeed a reversal of fortunes at Netherne and Mapperley, where the social conditions, after an initial improvement, returned to approximately their previous level. At both hospitals the process of clinical improvement was also reversed, and patients became more socially withdrawn. One cannot suppose that the curves representing social and clinical change, which move in phase with each other, but which show concomitant improvement and deterioration at different times in different hospitals, are describing the natural history of an illness.

The hypothesis that the social conditions under which a patient lives (particularly poverty of the social environment) are actually responsible for part of the symptomatology (particularly the negative symptoms), has been subjected to a number of fairly rigorous tests, any one of which it might well have failed; but it has not been disproved.

'Secondary' impairments: attitudes to discharge

A patient suffering from any chronic illness is liable to develop 'secondary' handicaps which do not arise directly out of the disease process, although they would not have occurred if he had remained well. There are two main types. In the first place, there is the patient's personal reaction to being ill, depending not only on the nature and severity of the disease, but on his previous personality, social attitudes, and experience of illness. Second, there is the reaction of the social groups, general and local, in which the patient plays a part, and upon whose goodwill his conditions of life may depend. If these two kinds of reaction are favourable, even a severe primary disability may not hinder a patient from achieving a successful resettlement. If they are adverse, even a mildly handicapped patient is likely to remain unsettled.

Once the patient is admitted to hospital, particularly if the chances of discharge are remote, the expectations of staff and other patients become paramount. The longer the patient stays, the less likely is he to practise everyday social roles and any ability that he originally had may atrophy from disuse. The patient, who originally has no intention of staying in hospital (Wing, *et al.* 1964), gradually changes his attitudes and eventually may not wish to leave (Wing 1961). 'Institutionalism' of this kind is a special case of the development of secondary handicaps.

In the present study there is a strong relationship between attitude to discharge and length of stay. The longer a patient has been in hospital the more likely he or she is to wish to stay or to be indifferent about leaving.

Unfavourable attitudes were very resistant to change. The social improvements brought about at the three hospitals – particularly those at Severalls – did not seem to do more than slow down the process whereby patients tend to adopt a wish to remain in hospital as they stay longer. Previous work on changing attitudes to work outside hospital, in long-stay patients with schizophrenia, showed that the most successful technique is a realistic course of preparation which demonstrates to patients, relatives, and staff that they do have the capability (Wing, Bennett, and Denham 1964). A planned system of travelling by public transport and other everyday activities, trial weekends and holidays with relatives or in hostels, is probably the best way to change attitudes to discharge in selected patients.

Of the twenty-three patients who were discharged by the time of the second survey in 1964, nineteen had had favourable attitudes when seen in 1960. Of the remaining thirty patients, who were outside hospital at the time of the final survey in January 1968, only twelve had wanted to leave in 1960, and a further five did so at the time of the latest survey before leaving. Thus thirteen patients either changed their minds later on, or were still doubtful when they did leave.

The nature of institutionalism in mental hospitals

Indifference about leaving lies at the very heart of institutionalism, and we would expect to find it developing in the inmates of most total institutions, particularly in those from vulnerable groups such as the physically handicapped, mentally retarded, or those with inadequate personalities. Schizophrenic patients are probably particularly at risk because of their vulnerability to social under-stimulation, which also contributes to the development of unfavourable attitudes. In long-stay patients, these elements – clinical and social poverty and 'institutionalism' – often occur together and it may then seem difficult to disentangle the elements. However, secondary impairment develops in patients who have only mild or moderate clinical symptoms the longer they stay in hospital. It is important to consider the primary and secondary disabilities separately because the treatments are different. We have seen that an increase in activity, which reduces social withdrawal and affective blunting, does not necessarily change attitudes. On the other hand, more personal possessions, a smarter hairstyle, and so on, do not necessarily lead to clinical change, though they would be expected to reduce secondary impairments. In severely-handicapped patients the first task is to bring about clinical improvement – but preventive work, to prevent deterioration in self-respect and self-confidence and to stop the development of institutionalized attitudes, is also needed. In moderately-handicapped patients the main task is to change attitudes, or to prevent them from becoming unfavourable.

Thus institutionalism in mental hospitals should be regarded as no different, in principle, from the condition that develops in other institutions, although it may be seen in its most severe form in long-stay schizophrenic patients.

The organization of social therapy in mental hospitals

The second part of this discussion will be devoted to a consideration of how the knowledge about social methods of treatment gained in this study may be applied. The first question to decide is which changes in social environment were most important in bringing about the clinical improvement.

Which social changes were most important?

Our analysis brings out quite clearly that the most important single factor associated with improvement of primary handicaps was a reduction in the amount of time doing nothing. There was a general improvement in the social environment of all patients, but it was much greater for those who were better clinically in 1964 and, above all, the amount of inactivity had markedly decreased. The only really important category distinguishing patients who improved clinically from those who did not was 'work and occupational therapy'. Although time spent watching television or listening to the radio or in various leisure occupations (a very diverse category) also increased, there was little to choose between the increase in patients who improved clinically and the increase in those who did not. More time was spent watching television or listening to the radio or in various leisure pursuits (knitting, talking, going for walks, etc) by those who improved clinically *and* by those who did not. It was probably the introduction of industrial work at Severalls which accounted for much of the clinical improvement there. Thus inactivity appears to be one of the greatest dangers for the chronic schizophrenic patient and seems to be directly responsible for a certain proportion of clinical symptomatology such as flatness of affect, poverty of speech, and social withdrawal.

However, ward restrictiveness also seems to play an independent part in promoting or maintaining negative symptoms. This may well be because a highly restrictive ward is under-stimulating even when patients are engaged in doing something – their activities are of a more habitual and less interesting kind.

The other social changes, such as increased contact with the outside world, a more optimistic mood among the nursing staff, and an increased supply of personal belongings, are less important so far as primary disabilities are concerned. They are nevertheless of major importance in reducing secondary handicaps. A woman with well-fitting clothes, pleasantly styled hair, and judiciously applied make-up, who spends most of her day working as a typist in the nurses' training school, who makes expeditions to the local shops when she wishes to, and patronizes the town cinema with her friend, is far removed from the stereotype of the 'back ward' schizophrenic; and the attitudes of staff and relatives, as well as her own attitudes to herself, depend in large measure on this 'front' that she is able to show to the world. The same patient, in Kerry Ward in 1960, presented quite a different image, one which would have confirmed the gloomy views which used to be common currency among those who thought they knew about the course of schizophrenia.

Clearly, these changes have to be brought about gradually; and when there are limited resources, certain patients will receive attention at the expense of others. Thus, at Severalls, the restrictiveness of the ward regimes did not decrease very remarkably over all although the social conditions in the wards, and the social experiences of many patients, did improve considerably. Similarly, in the American hospital, there was very high restrictiveness combined with relatively low morbidity. The creation of a liberal regime in which the patients could participate fully according to their ability is, however, an important step in their resocialization and a more economical way of achieving part of it. The major lesson to be drawn is that general social changes are no substitute for specific social treatment aimed at each individual, and based upon a detailed knowledge of his handicaps. The two approaches are complementary.

We did not attempt to measure self-attitudes in patients in this series, but we would certainly suggest that they improved, in so far as they reflected the new social status that many people were able to attain. They were, however, still in hospital, and more specific measures to change the whole atmosphere away from that of an institution towards those of commoner social groups – in particular the family – had not proceeded very far except at Netherne (and, even there, only for a small proportion of the patients in our series). These were traditional environments, removing many of those elements which had disfigured them in the custodial era, but not radically reforming their social structures. One would not expect profound changes in attitudes to discharge or to work, under these circumstances.

The organization necessary to bring about clinical improvement

The organization of the patient's day in Longfield Villa may be taken as the model towards which all three hospitals were striving and which Netherne came closest to attaining. Ideally, patients should do things for themselves; get up, get their meals, do the chores, go to work, spend their leisure time, and organize their way of life, as they would if they were not in hospital and not handicapped. This means a constant testing to see whether the time has come for a particular function to be actively taken over by a patient rather than being passively exercised by a helper. Left to himself, the severely-handicapped schizophrenic patient lapses into inactivity. With active supervision this tendency is counteracted – but for how long need the active supervision be kept up? When can it be relaxed? These are some of the essential questions of social treatment (Wing and Freudenberg 1961) and they may be more easily answered if staff and patients can share experiences in regular group sessions.

Underlying the policy at all three hospitals was the assumption that specialized environments should be created for various categories of patient. Thus Longfield Villa was set up for the most severely handicapped patients, while Downswood catered for patients who were able to participate in life outside hospital to a certain extent and for whom there was a fair prospect of discharge in the relatively near future. At Mapperley there were wards run by the patients themselves, with only an experienced part-time staff member to keep an eye on things. At Netherne there was a range of industrial workshops catering for patients with different levels of handicap. Netherne provided the greatest variety of environments within the hospital, but both Mapperley and Severalls adopted the principle.

Thus from the intimate level of the ward nurse or occupational therapist engaged in helping a schizophrenic patient to function in a social environment, to the more distant level of hospital planning of specialized workshops and wards, the intention was to provide specific treatment for specific individuals.

This work contains lessons for social therapy in social settings other than mental hospitals, as the focus of care shifts more and more to alternative environments. Not only can it be demonstrated that the social treatments carried out by mental hospital staff do have value and that the course of schizophrenic illnesses can be influenced in hospital, as it can outside, but there is a salutary reminder that efforts must be kept up and that reform itself has a natural history. New forms of community agency must be developed in which the best aspects of the mental hospital tradition are preserved even if the buildings themselves are not. The services provided by the various specialized social environments of the good mental hospital are still needed. The experience of the rehabilitation team is relevant to the new problems of community psychiatry. If these skills and traditions are lost it will be a long time before they are developed again. Rehabilitation remains one of the most necessary, as well as one of the most rewarding, aspects of psychiatry, and its scientific basis is beginning to unite biological, psychological, and social researches in a way which may prove a model for other fields of medicine. The present ferment of change provides an opportunity for further progress but only if the lessons of the past – particularly the state of 'community care' which preceded the foundation of the early hospitals for 'moral treatment' – are remembered and profitably used.

24 Alienation and the social structure: case analysis of a hospital

*Rose Laub Coser**

[*This paper has been edited from the original according to the editors' strategy. The author is Professor at the Health Sciences Center and in the Sociology Department of the State University of New York at Stony Brook.*]

This paper sets out to specify some mechanisms through which 'the social structure operates to exert pressure upon individuals for one or another of alternative modes of behavior'. (Merton 1957.)

Sunnydale Hospital, a community hospital on the outskirts of the industrial center of Maplewood in the western United States, provides a good opportunity for studying the relation between selected kinds of behavior and social structure. Sunnydale's 650 beds, occupied by patients who are said not to be capable of improvement, are distributed over five buildings. One hundred additional beds are located in a sixth building, which is the Rehabilitation Center for patients with polio, respiratory, muscular, rheumatic, and other diseases requiring intensive rehabilitation programmes. The social structure of the Center and the

*extracted from chapter 8, in Eliot Freidson (ed.), *The Hospital in Modern Society* (1964) New York: The Free Press: 231–65

attitudes of its staff will be compared with the structure and attitudes of Sunnydale proper. The data are derived from structured interviews with twenty-seven registered nurses (out of a total of thirty registered nurses of the day shift), focussed interviews with ten interns, participant observation, and from systematic observation in all wards of the interaction between staff and patients and of staff members among themselves.

Alienation

The definition of the situation

The different goal orientations of the two types of wards are recognized by all the registered nurses interviewed. At least once during the interview, all Center nurses mentioned the goal of restoring patients to the community, whereas none of the Sunnydale nurses ever did so. The different orientations are based in large part on the nature of the illness of the patients. Three of Sunnydale's buildings are assigned to 'custodial' cases; these give the 'stamp' to the hospital in spite of the fact that two of its buildings are said to consist of 'active treatment' wards, one for acute and one for long-term patients. Moreover, in the opinion of physicians both at Sunnydale and at the Center – though generally Sunnydale's patients are defined as 'terminal' or 'custodial' – a number of Sunnydale's patients could be rehabilitated. In spite of the fact that Sunnydale's patient population is not homogeneous in regard to prognosis, the nurses refer to their hospital in such terms as, 'This is only an old people's home as far as I am concerned', or, 'This is considered the end of the road, and people here talk of them as vegetables'. On the other hand, the Center, whose patients are being prepared for a return to the community, also has patients whose illness is irreversible. For example, in a discussion about a terminal case at the Center, a physician impatiently retorted to the objection that the patient knew she had at most five years to live, 'We all have to die'. He remarked that if we let the therapy program be guided by such considerations, we 'may as well have a concentration camp instead of a hospital'. Thus, despite differences between wards as well as individual differences within the wards, in both environments all patients tend to be regarded *as if* they fit the respective goal, whether or not they actually do.

The stated goal, then, provides the definition of the situation. What is considered disruptive in one situation is considered rewarding in the other. If patients are defined as 'terminal and custodial', plans to discharge them can be seen as disrupting activities. Several Sunnydale nurses say that they prefer a low turnover of patients 'because of the type of help we have' or because 'there's too much desk work' involved in discharging and admitting patients. One nurse explains that 'the doctor will listen to me' if she feels that the patient should not be discharged because 'if they do get discharged and come back in a week or two, it's more trouble in work and time'. She adds: 'You like the same patients in the same beds instead of having all the book work that is necessitated by changes.'

Center nurses do not make such comments. Where the goal is to restore patients to the community, discharge becomes gratifying, as indicated by the following: 'On this unit we have the satisfaction of getting patients discharged out of the hospital; nurses really get satisfaction if a patient comes in hemiplegic and then is discharged home walking within a few months.' Discharge of patients at the Center is seen as reward for achievement. When such rewards cannot be expected, work is not seen as a means of achievement but as 'a job to be done'.

Evidence concerning the differing orientations of Sunnydale and Center nurses comes from the responses to two questions that were asked in the interview: the first asked the nurses' judgment about their site of work, the other, their perception of needs for the future. In their answers to both questions, Sunnydale nurses are means-oriented in contrast to Center nurses, who are goal-oriented.

In answer to the question 'How would you describe a ward when it's looking at its best?' Sunnydale nurses are more likely than Center nurses to stress the physical appearance of the ward (sixteen out of seventeen as compared with one out of ten nurses at Center), indicating that housekeeping problems stand in the foreground of attention. The following is a typical Sunnydale description of 'a ward at its best': 'When it is finished and you stand at the head of the ward and look in, it is beautifully done, everything is clean.' Nine of the Center nurses, in contrast, respond by referring to the behaviour of patients, a concern to be expected among those who pursue the goal of restoring patients to the community. The following is a typical answer from the Center: 'I like to see everybody out of bed and as active as possible. I like a certain amount of, not humour, but at least cheerful informal ward setting.'

The emphasis by Sunnydale nurses on physical aspects in contrast to the emphasis on human achievement in the Center is consistent with perceptions of future needs. Asked 'What are the most important things needed in your ward?', Sunnydale nurses emphasize physical improvements to facilitate work and efficiency; some of the Center nurses who want physical improvements explain that their purpose is to benefit patients. Center nurses are also more likely to stress the need for better personal relations among the staff or between staff and patients.

Clearly, work has a different meaning at Sunnydale, where attention is focussed on shortage of personnel, paper work, or other routine. In contrast to the *organic* conception of work, in which concern is with human implications, is the *ritualistic* conception of work, where focus is on 'dead matter' and work is *mechanical*. As one nurse so cogently explained: 'Well, my dear, I don't know. There isn't anything that I find unpleasant. *I have done it so long, I just automatically do it*' (italics supplied).

Involvement in work

Sunnydale nurses are not deeply involved in their work. Although they don't dislike it much, neither do they have important reasons for liking it. When asked about their feelings, they reply by referring to routine matters. But Center nurses seem to have strong feelings about the sources of gratification as well as of frustration.

Asked 'What do you like least in your work?' most Sunnydale nurses mention some routine as a source of dissatisfaction, such as 'I don't like removing impactions'. Furthermore, their references to sources of dissatisfaction are not expressed with much effect. The first impression upon interviewing Sunnydale nurses is that if there are any dissatisfactions, they do not concern professional issues. The example given by the nurses' director of Sunnydale illustrates this point: 'There are not a great many grievances. A year ago they had complaints about the parking situation; they had to park the cars too far from the buildings. So now we've changed that.'

In contrast, the complaints of Center nurses tend to show concern with professional relations and professional issues (eight out of ten nurses at Center, but none of the seventeen nurses at Sunnydale). These nurses tend to 'dislike most' conflicts among the staff or certain conditions of the patients: 'The thing I like least is the stress I feel when we have such a tremendous working organization and we can't communicate to get the job done.' Or again, when 'some patients get exasperated'. These typical statements also suggest both presence and awareness of strong feelings – 'The stress I feel' or 'patients get exasperated'.

Sunnydale nurses tend to answer in general rather than in concrete terms; they like 'the care of humanity' or 'nursing care'. One nurse implies that her gratification stems from being able to get away from work: 'It's a well-rounded day ... The employees can put in requests for vacation.' In contrast, the majority of Center nurses derive satisfaction from professional achievements, and express their feelings about them. One nurse, typical of the others, says that she likes best 'taking someone who is crippled or injured and showing them the means so that they can be self-sufficient, and seeing them accomplish it. It's a tremendous challenge.'

Self-image

Hughes (Hughes 1958:43) suggests that when you ask people what work they do, they are likely to answer in terms of 'who they are'; that is, they attempt to establish and validate their own identity by referring to the identity of their work in a publicly recognized and preferably esteemed occupational or professional category. My interviews with nurses, however, suggest that not all of them give such self-enhancing descriptions of 'who they are' when asked 'What is the most important thing you do?' Although many of them give a broad, inclusive description of the nature of their work, such as 'problem-solving' or 'helping patients reach their goal', others give simple concrete descriptions of tasks such as 'keep patients clean' or 'watch for symptoms'. This suggests two different types of orientation to work. Some nurses refer to some concrete part of what they do; others develop a more inclusive conception of their occupational roles.

The data suggest that most Center nurses refer to their inclusive role (nine out of ten Center nurses compared with two out of seventeen Sunnydale nurses), while Sunnydale nurses are more likely to refer to some specific task. This would suggest that when Hughes says work is one of the most important parts of a person's social identity, he refers to one type of work and one type of person; he speaks of relatively unalienated work and relatively unalienated people.

The connection between conception of work role and the perception of the social field is highlighted in the drawings the nurses were asked to make of 'a nurse at work'. Eight nurses drew a picture of a nurse without a patient; one of these nurses was at the Center, the other seven were at Sunnydale.

All nurses deriving their work satisfaction from achievement who drew a picture, make the patient a part of their image of 'a nurse at work', and so do most nurses who derive their satisfaction from professional relations. But none of the nurses who speak of their satisfaction in terms of general care have their drawings depict work as part of a social arrangement. Six nurses, one from Sunnydale and five from the Center, focus their attention on better staff relations or on better care of patients when describing needed improvements: all these include a patient in their drawings of a 'nurse at work'. The data support the hypothesis that a worker's alienation from his work is associated with his alienation from those with whom he is associated in his occupational role.

Melvin Seeman (Seeman 1959) has identified five alternative meanings in which Marx's concept of alienation is used in sociological writings. He distinguishes between powerlessness, meaninglessness, normlessness, self-estrangement, and isolation. These are, of course, not always empirically distinct in all situations. At Sunnydale, all these elements are present and interrelated. Sunnydale nurses are alienated because they are *powerless* to implement a significant goal. Unable to obtain gratifying results from their work, they find it *meaningless* and so cannot use it to fashion a meaningful self-image. Not being able to express their social identity in their work, they are *self-estranged* in the work situation. Consequently, they become estranged from their social field and see themselves as *isolated* individuals. It will become clear in what follows that Sunnydale nurses work under conditions that also isolate them physically from other professional groups – a condition that contributes to the *normlessness* of behavior in the form of retreatism. *Alienation*, it seems, is a *syndrome* composed of all the elements that Seeman has carefully defined.

Deviation from professional norms

An acute shortage of personnel does not necessarily increase each person's load; it may get so bad that it legitimizes withdrawal from the task. At Sunnydale, abandoning the prestigious goal of recovery results also in abandoning some professionally prescribed means of medical practice. A nurses' supervisor illustrates this point: 'The intern would go through the charts on his day and never change the prescriptions; sometimes he would just add to the old prescriptions, and *we* can't change them.' At Sunnydale, interns as well as nurses seem to retreat from what is usually called professional behavior.

Not only do interns withdraw from the wards; more important still, nurses and interns help each other to maintain this type of withdrawal. Physicians do not interfere in the active treatment ward when the buzzers at the beds of patients are disconnected and the electric cord tied up so that patients cannot connect it themselves. In turn, nurses know that if they 'call [a doctor] without too much need he doesn't like it', and consequently they are, in the praiseful words of one intern, 'outstanding [since they are] ultraconservative in calling the doctor'. Another intern thinks that the nurses are not always reliable since, as he explains, 'they sometimes call for minor things'. In this case it seems that the competence of the nurse is measured not so much by her achievements as by her willingness to help the doctor to stand aside. Thus, where sanctions are at work at Sunnydale, they often press for the evasion of norms. It is partly on this basis that some consensus between doctors and nurses is established.

Consequently, Sunnydale is characterized by a lack of those inter-professional conflicts described by observers in other hospitals. But lack of conflict is not necessarily functional for an organization. As in this case, it may be a result of relative withdrawal from the task. One nurse in an active treatment ward explains that she has little difficulty with doctors: '[I have] very little contact with interns. They go their own way.' Not only are there too few physicians to be 'underfoot' – a frequent accusation in other hospitals – and not only do they stay too short a time for strong sentiments, either positive or negative, to develop, but the interaction between nurses and physicians is greatly curbed by both professional groups encouraging mutual avoidance. It appears that avoid-ance is a means for adapting to tasks that seem to be deprived of a meaningful goal.

Affirmation of professional norms

The social structure of the Center offers a contrast sufficient to highlight some structural determinants of alienation. The staff there is character-ized by its multiple professional affiliations, and mechanisms have evolved that assure a large measure of social control. The various pro-fessional groups work next to each other, with each other, and often in competition with each other.

As we have known ever since Durkheim, the interdependence of various occupations resulting from the division of labor brings about the 'organic solidarity' that helps hold modern society together. Organic solidarity consists of involvement with one another of interdependent status occupants. They are bound by common interests, though they may be in conflict regarding the means for implementing these interests. In some settings, such as the Center, they can observe one another at close quarters, and all are under pressure to orient themselves to differential expectations in these complex criss-crossing circles. Persons of various status positions and different professional orientations and expectations are held together by their common commitment to the concrete goal of returning patients to the community; there is strong concern on everyone's part with achievement and failure. And precisely because of such zeal, conflicts do arise. All nurses in the Center report difficulties with doctors, whereas only a third of the nurses at Sunnydale do so. As one nurse explains: 'Everybody feels that they like to be in charge of the situation. Everybody says, "This is my business", and nobody gets an over-all picture.'

Fighting over controversial issues is considered legitimate [at the Center]. Differences of opinion and expectation are dealt with at regular and frequent all-staff meetings or smaller conferences. These provide a patterned opportunity for the carrying out of conflicts between the different professional groups, which continuously recall the goal to be pursued and the norms that should govern behavior. Meetings provide an occasion for reaffirming the goal and formulating norms, and also bring onto the level of rational discourse and instrumental behavior feelings that without such a forum might become laden with affect. The open expressions of opinions and judgments give a professional definition to personal involvement. This is especially important in an atmosphere of deep involvements since these could give rise to a clash of personalities; but since antagonisms are recognized, conflicts at the Center tend to be limited to the functionally specific task at hand. Instead of being a sign of social disorganization they are expressions of, as well as means for, social control among various professional groups and individuals.

Social control is reinforced by the fact that the meetings provide institutionalized settings for *observability* among persons of various fields of specialization and in various positions in the hierarchy. At the same time, they largely limit the time and place of observability, thus assuring a patterned measure of insulation. We need not belabor the point that if persons variously located in the social structure are to evaluate the behavior of others, they must at regular intervals either see one another behave or at least be in a position to obtain information about their behavior. If such information is lacking, status occupants become exempted from the judgment of competent colleagues, and role perform-ance may sink below tolerable standards. While some insulation from observability is also needed so that persons can go about their work without unpredicted interference by role partners with whom they stand in an authority relationship, at Sunnydale, isolation of nurses from pro-fessional colleagues and the scarcity of interaction with other professionals eliminate a source of information and social control as well.

Indeed, conferences and meetings do more than provide information about professional behavior. They also make status occupants aware of the differing expectations held by role partners significant to them. As a result, persons in different positions are helped to articulate their roles and to formulate a professional self-image.

A further property of social structure that facilitates articulation of the nurses' roles at the Center is the presence of a sufficiently large number of registered nurses in one unit. Every nurse knows that she is not alone in facing contradictory expectations of many role partners. They can therefore articulate their roles *collectively*.

Both the fact that all nurses share the same difficulties and that there are avenues for verbalizing them make it possible for these issues to be removed from the level of 'personal problems' to that of social organization. The nurses are in a position not so much to discuss their 'personal problems' as to articulate their *professional* role.

At the Center, then, the very conditions and mechanisms that provide a source of social control – multiplicity of role partners, conflicts among professional groups, mutual observability, as well as its limitation, and the regular meetings to deal with these – also provide the conditions for the articulation of roles and formation of professional self-images.

These conditions do not prevail at Sunnydale because (1) the goal of caring for patients, as it is understood, restricts the staff's task primarily to problems of housekeeping, and (2) social arrangements are such that status occupants suffer from a restricted role set, that is, from a restriction of the number of significant role partners.

With too much work to do, everyone is more concerned with specific problems of housekeeping than with problems concerning either staff relations or more remote goals. The understaffing of Sunnydale's wards is, to a large extent, a result of the definition of 'custodial care': given this goal orientation, the composition of the population – patients as well as staff – is geared to the definition of this goal.

Under these conditions, a goal that does not seem 'worthy' (interns tend to say that it isn't 'worthwhile' to spend much energy on 'these' patients) and an overwhelming work load, the few people who are in potentially responsible positions tend to withdraw. This keeps them from being informed about the norms and behavior of others. Also, they are not motivated to seek information about them, since prevailing conditions seem to make it impossible for them to use the information effectively.

With too few professional persons available, few professions represented, and the tendency of the few available persons to withdraw, status occupants at Sunnydale suffer from a *restricted role set*, that is, from a restriction of the number of role partners. This has the following consequences: (*a*) Sunnydale nurses (as well as all other status occupants at Sunnydale) work under conditions of *low exposure to observability* – a condition that results in the reduction of social control; (*b*) since there are few persons *differentially* located in the social structure, there are hardly any conflicting expectations faced by status occupants;

therefore they are not required to be *continuously engaged in articulating their roles in relation to the members of their role sets* and consequently forming a professional self-image; (*c*) given their scarcity, registered nurses are relatively deprived of role partners occupying the *same* status position as themselves, so that there is little opportunity for them to articulate collectively, as professionals, the responsibilities and limitations of the relationships they share.

The scaling down of the goal of recovery of the sick not only has the direct consequence of inducing the staff to adopt ritualistic or retreatist behavior. By restricting the number of role partners for status occupants in responsible positions – an organizational restriction that is a further consequence of the scaling down of the goal – it provides the structural setting for patterned non-conformity as well as institutionalization of the alienation syndrome.

PART VIII
Social causes of disease

25 Depression: a sociological view

*George W. Brown**

*[This paper is complete, with the addition of the three tables.
The author is Professor of Sociology in the UK.]*

I have been asked for a personal statement about depression. Of all
psychiatric conditions depression is perhaps the most fitting for a
sociologist to study. It is an affliction of a person's sense of values;
and an exploration of the way people give meaning to their world can
be expected to throw some light on a condition whose central feature,
in Aaron Beck's (1967) terms, is a feeling that there is no meaning in
the world, that the future is hopeless, and the self worthless. Around
this three-fold sense of futility cluster different psychological and somatic
symptoms none of which on their own are either sufficient or necessary
for the diagnosis. But I will leave this aside and start at the heart of
the matter – with aetiology.

I believe that depression is essentially a social phenomenon. (If this
were not a personal statement I would say that present evidence does
not make it unreasonable to hold this view.) I would not make the same
claim for schizophrenia, though its onset and course are also greatly

*from the *Bethlem and Maudsley Gazette* (1977): 9–12, Summer

influenced by social factors. Society and depression are more fundamentally linked. I can envisage societies where depression is absent and
others where the majority suffer from depression. While this is social
science fiction something not too unlike it has been documented. At
least a quarter of working-class women with children living in London
suffer from a depressive disorder which, if they were to present themselves at an out-patient clinic, psychiatrists would accept as clinical
depression; while women with children living in crofting households
in the Outer Hebrides are practically free of depression no matter what
their social class. (They do experience more anxiety conditions, but I
believe that this is another story.) Moreover, I know of no compelling
reason to believe that the many bodily correlates of depression such
as those revealed by work on bioamines are any more than the *result*
of social and psychological factors. This is not to deny the possible
aetiological implications of recent biochemical research, nor the possible
aetiological role of genetic and constitutional factors. But taking account
of the need to explain differences in the rate of depression in whole
populations, I do not think that there is likely to be any more than
a very modest primary aetiological influence from biochemical processes,
that is, from such processes alone. The evidence for such a primary role
for psychological and social factors is certainly far more convincing.

Like most doing research in the field of depression I am firmly
convinced of a multifactorial view: that factors at many levels can play
a role in aetiology. But this perspective should not disguise the need
to establish the *relative* contribution of the various levels. Lip-service
tends to be given to a multifactorial view but often in practice, in teaching,
in research, and in clinical work only a single class of factor is seriously
considered. Ritual obeisance to many variables allows pursuit of one.
A psychiatrist in 1967 who asserted that a woman attending his clinic
could not be clinically depressed as her condition was clearly related
to her bad housing was perhaps expressing in a somewhat unsophisticated
way the same views as many of his colleagues. Clinicians understandably
desire research that will justify intervention in clinical settings. They
also want theories that would be both intellectually challenging and serve
as a basis for their claims to professional expertise within medicine.
The failure of sociological ideas and methods to make much of an impact
on psychiatric teaching has meant that most psychiatrists see little
intellectual challenge in a sociological approach concentrating on the
current environment. This also means that many have remained tied
to a narrow view of science in which only experimentation is given full
honours.

Of course, during the last two decades there has been important changes not least due to the lead of Sir Aubrey Lewis. But social psychiatry still needs to devote more of its time to the heady and dangerous job of causal analysis in natural settings; only in this way is it likely to get the necessary challenge and impetus to develop measures and methods that will have the authority to influence psychiatry as a whole.

During the last eight years my colleagues and I have done our best to follow such a path: our ideas about depression cannot be said to diverge all that much from ideas expressed *somewhere* in the psychiatric literature. (Has any other discipline speculated quite so much?) Any claim to originality probably mainly rests on the way factors have been brought together in a causal model; and any claims to attention on the consideration we have given to methodological problems. Indeed the model is sufficiently well based for some interest to be shown in the theory that we have linked to it. But in what follows, model and theory should be kept distinct; claims made for our causal model cannot be made for our more speculative theory.

The job of creating such a model involves developing measures and research design so that a claim can be made that the factors, following the temporal order set out in the model (*Figure 11* see over), are *in some way* involved in bringing about depression. Obvious biases must be ruled out and objections that would trivialize the model must be met. (For example, while life-events do play a causal role they merely bring about a depressive disorder that would have occurred before long in any case without any pre-event occurring.) We have made some progress; certain kinds of severe life-events and difficulties do appear to bring about the majority of depressive disorders – both among women treated by psychiatrists and among women found to be depressed after being selected at random from the general population (see *Table 33*).

Table 33   *Proportion with at least one severely threatening event or at least one major difficulty in the period before onset for patients and onset cases or interviews for 'normal' and 'borderline' women*

	patients $(N = 114)$ %	onset cases $(N = 37)$ %	'normal' and 'borderline' women $(N = 382)$ %
1 severe event alone	30 ⎫	41 ⎫	13 ⎫
2 severe event and major difficulty	32 ⎬ 75	24 ⎬ 89	6 ⎬ 30
3 major difficulty	14 ⎭	24 ⎭	11 ⎭
4 no severe event or major difficulty	25	11	70

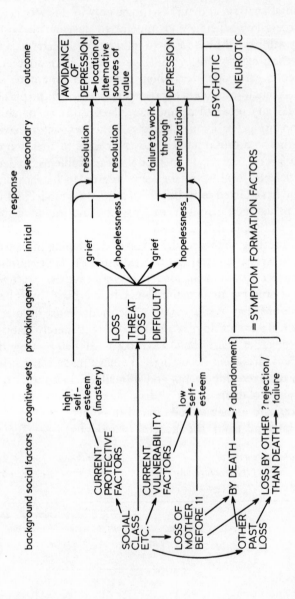

Figure 11 (*key*: CAPITALS = Causal model)

The kind of depression does not matter: these *provoking agents* are as strongly associated with the onset of psychotic as neurotic depressive conditions. Perhaps the most challenging claim of the model is that provoking agents (i.e., events and difficulties) are rarely sufficient to bring about depression – although they do determine *when* the disorders occur.

This is best illustrated by the way depression is linked to social class. Working-class women in London are not only far more likely to suffer from depression, they are also far more likely to develop a clear depressive disorder in the presence of a major life-event or difficulty (see *Table 34*). Something other than the provoking agent is at work.

Table 34 *Percentage of women developing a psychiatric disorder (i.e., caseness) in year by life-stage, social class, and whether preceded by a severe event or major difficulty (chronic cases excluded)*

	severe event/ major difficulty %	no severe event/ major difficulty %
women without child at home		
middle class	22 (7/32)	0 (0/62)
working class	10 (3/30)	2 (1/44)
women with child at home		
middle class	8 (3/36)	1 (1/80)
working class	31 (21/67)	1 (1/68)
all women		
middle class	15 (10/68)	1 (1/142)
working class	25 (24/97)	3 (2/112)

There is in fact a second set of factors. If a woman does not have an intimate relationship with a husband or boyfriend – one in which she feels she can confide and trust – she is much more likely to break down in the presence of a major life-event or difficulty. Similarly she is also at greater risk if she has three or more children under fifteen at home, if she is unemployed, and if she lost her mother (but not father) before the age of eleven. We call these *vulnerability factors* – although more optimistically they can be seen in a reverse way and called protective factors. None are capable of producing depression on their own, but they greatly increase chances of breakdown in the presence of a provoking agent. (*Table 35* see over.) Some of the social class difference is explained by the fact that working class women in London experience more untoward life-events and difficulties – in this sense their lives are much tougher. But most of the class difference is due to their excess of vulnerability factors which put working-class women at risk for depression at the time of a major life-event or difficulty. The low rate of depression in the Outer Hebrides is probably due to the much greater degree of protection their culture and society gives these women – but this has still to be documented in detail.

Table 35 *Proportion of women developing psychiatric disorder in the year among women who experienced a severe event or major difficulty by vulnerability factors (intimacy, employment status, early loss of mother and 3+ children under 15 at home)*

		with event or difficulty			without event or difficulty		
'a'* intimacy relationship regardless	employed	(4/53)	9%	} (9/88) *10%*	(1/117)	1%	} (2/193) *1%*
	not employed	(5/45)	11%		(1/76)	1%	
non-'a'* intimacy relationship excluding early loss of mother or 3+ children under 15 living at home	employed	(6/39)	15%		(0/34)	0%	
	not employed	(7/23)	30%		(2/19)	11%	
non-'a'* intimacy relationship with early loss of mother or 3+ children under 15 living at home	employed	(5/8)	63%		(0/7)	0%	
	not employed	(6/6)	100%		(0/2)	0%	
		(33/164)	20%		(4/255)	2%	

* essentially an 'a' intimacy relationship is one where the respondent reports a confiding relationship (where both partners can talk to each other about any personal matter) and this person is either a man or a member of the respondent's household

Recently a third factor has been added to this model. While only loss of a mother before eleven increases the risk of a woman developing depression, other past losses of close relatives, largely in childhood and adolescence, influence the type and severity of depression. We call these *symptom formation* factors. Loss by *death* is strongly associated with psychotic-like depressive symptoms and the severity and *loss by other means* (e.g., parents separating) to neurotic-like depressive symptoms (and their severity). Only loss of mother before eleven plays two roles – as a vulnerability factor increasing risk of depression and as a symptom formation factor. Otherwise past loss merely determines the form and severity of a depressive disorder once it has occurred.

This is a rough outline of the model – stated without necessary caveats. But what does it all mean? What about theory? Consider employment and its protective role for women. Is it because it improves her economic circumstances, alleviates her boredom, keeps her occupied, brings her a greater variety of social contacts, or enhances her sense of personal worth? And just why should any of these aspects play a protective role? A causal model is not enough: theory is needed to explain what is happening. Theory unfortunately takes longer than a causal model to develop and to test. Any theory concerning the aetiology of depression has to deal with two crucial 'facts' provided by our model. First, that on the whole provoking life-events mainly involve major losses (if this term is allowed a certain licence to include events such as learning of a husband's infidelity); major difficulties and threats of loss can also at times bring about a depressive disorder. Something more than loss must be involved. Second, in the absence of a vulnerability factor such provoking agents rarely bring about depression. In other words, no matter how catastrophic a loss depression will not follow without the presence of at least one vulnerability factor.

We have speculated that low self-esteem is the common feature behind all four vulnerability factors and it is this that makes sense of our results. It is not loss itself that is important but the capacity of a woman to hope for better things once an event or difficulty has occurred. In response to a provoking agent relatively specific feelings of hopelessness are likely to occur: the person has usually lost an important source of value – something that may have been derived from a person, a role, or an idea. If this develops into a *general* feeling of hopelessness it may form the central feature of the depressive disorder itself; and Beck's (1967) triad of cognitions accompanies the well known affective and somatic symptoms of depression. Essential in any such generalization of hopelessness is a woman's ongoing self-esteem, her sense of her ability to control her world, and her confidence that alternative sources of value will be available. If the woman's self-esteem is low *before* the onset of any depression she will be less likely to be able to see herself as emerging from her privation. And, of course, once depression has occurred feelings of confidence and self-worth can sink even lower.

It must not be overlooked that an appraisal of general hopelessness may be entirely realistic: the future for many women *is* bleak. But given an event or difficulty, low self-esteem will increase the chances of such an interpretation of hopelessness. Here inner and outer worlds meet, and internal and external resources come together. And from there the sociologist must go on to build links with the wider cultural, economic, and political systems. Psychiatry cannot rest in the consulting room or even within the confines of a person's immediate social circle. Study of self-esteem cannot stop at the borders of a woman's personal world. For instance, may not feelings of low self-worth have something to do with the fact women are not paid for what many see as their central tasks? Do we take work seriously if it is not paid? The bitterness created by the recent attempts at wage control in all strata of male society suggest that more than economic considerations are involved in payment for work in our society.

While I have emphasized the role of the current environment our own results make it clear that this should not be taken too far – it is intended as a corrective. We carry with us our pasts. But I would again emphasize cognitive factors in explaining the effect of past loss. Loss of a mother before eleven, for instance, can be linked to the learning of uncontrollability, and through this to low self-esteem. Martin Seligman's (1975) concept of learned helplessness has got a good deal in common with the way we have interpreted the role of vulnerability and protective factors. But unlike him I see no reason to restrict our model to so-called 'reactive' or 'neurotic' depressive conditions. The various vulnerability factors increase the risk of all types of depression; for example, among our patients those with neurotic-like depressive symptoms were no more likely to have more vulnerability factors or provoking agents than those with psychotic symptoms; we also have seen that past loss in childhood and adolescence can greatly influence the much later expression of psychotic or neurotic symptoms.

Here again I would emphasize a cognitive interpretation – in this instance, concerning long held perceptions of abandonment for psychotic as against rejection and failure for neurotic depressive symptoms.

But this is particularly speculative and I have at this point pursued our theoretical ideas enough. I will just finally add that we have also argued for a second, but less important, aetiological mechanism in which self-esteem is again implicated. Low self-esteem can inhibit a woman carrying out the necessary grief work after a major loss – and complications leading to depression are then likely to arise. This would also make it more difficult for her to take advantage of alternative sources of value that might be available.

It is probably unnecessary to make the obvious point that these processes will have biological correlates. It is also possible that certain occurrences (e.g., early loss of mother, a depressive illness) may lead to more or less irreversible biochemical changes in the brain, thereby perhaps changing the mechanism of reward for the individual.

I am conscious of many gaps. I would have liked to explore the convergence of ideas about depression. There is, for instance, clearly a parallel between our sources of positive value and the psychologist's 'reinforcers' (e.g., Liberman and Raskin 1971), the psychoanalyst's 'narcissistic supplies' (e.g., Fenichel 1946) and the social scientist's concern with 'meaning' (e.g., Becker 1962). I am also aware of my failure to deal with the perennial issue of diagnosis. Some psychiatrists may wish to dispute the label of depressive psychiatric disorder we have given to women in the community – very few of whom were receiving psychiatric help. I would point out that this is likely to place psychiatry in a perplexing intellectual and ethical dilemma. The women do not appear to differ in any essential way from many seen and treated in out-patient clinics. Is a psychiatric label to be restricted to those who manage to present themselves in such clinics? Fresh ideas and new research are required to clarify this issue. Another topic which needs much more exploration is the boundary between normal grief and depression.

But most of all I am conscious of my failure to convey in human terms what I believe to be involved in depression and in avoiding depression. I comfort myself that the reader of the *Bethlem and Maudsley Gazette* least requires such an account. But, if my talk of value resources, provoking agents, vulnerability factors, and protective factors has not lost you, Shakespeare may be able to illustrate our theory and to suggest the power of alternative sources of value to rescue a person from the onset of depression.

'When in disgrace with Fortune and men's eyes,
I all alone beweep my outcast state,
And trouble deaf heaven with my bootless cries,
And look upon my self and curse my fate,
Wishing me like to one more rich in hope,
Featured like him, like him with friends possessed,
Desiring this man's art, and that man's scope.
With what I most enjoy contented least,
Yet in these thoughts my self almost despising,
Haply I think on thee, and then my state,
(Like to the lark at break of day arising

From sullen earth) sings hymns at heaven's gate,
For thy sweet love remembered such wealth brings,
That then I scorn to change my state with kings.'

(Sonnet XXIX)

26 Coronary heart disease in the western collaborative group study: final follow-up experience of eight and one-half years

Ray H. Rosenman, Richard J. Brand,
C. David Jenkins, Meyer Friedman,
Reuben Straus, & Moses Wurm*

[*This paper has been edited from the original according to the editors' general strategy except that space has been saved by cutting out a discussion of the differential relationship of the predictive factors to the different types of coronary heart disease. The authors are distinguished American physicians, psychologists, and biostaticians.*]

Methods and materials

The Western Collaborative Group Study (WCGS) was initiated in 1960–61 as a prospective epidemiological investigation of CHD incidence in 3,524 men, aged thirty-nine to fifty-nine years at intake, and employed in ten California companies. The methodology has been described in previous reports (Rosenman, *et al.* 1964; Rosenman, *et al.* 1970). Comprehensive data were obtained at intake and annually until the study was terminated, providing eight to nine years of follow-up, at which time a sufficient incidence of CHD had occurred as to make it unlikely that further follow-up would provide additional significant information. The intake studies were accomplished over an eighteen-month period from June 1960 to December 1961. Annual resurveys were done during the calendar twelve-month period, ending in December 1969, during which time the subjects were studied in order of intake, with minor

* extracted from the *Journal of the American Medical Association*, (1975) **233** (8): 872–77

exceptions. Excluded from longitudinal analyses were seventy-eight men under or over specified intake ages, 141 subjects with CHD manifest at intake, 106 employees of one firm that excluded itself from follow-up, and forty-five subjects who were lost to the study because of early relocation, non-CHD death, or self-exclusion prior to the first follow-up. This left 3,154 initially well subjects at risk for CHD. Manifest CHD occurred in 257 subjects during the follow-up period, and death occurred in 140 subjects: thirty-one of their initial CHD event, nineteen of a recurring CHD event, and ninety of non-CHD causes, including seven subjects who had developed manifest CHD. The remaining subjects were considered to be non-CHD cases, including 2,391 subjects who were examined throughout the entire period of follow-up and 423 subjects who were variously lost to follow-up. The death rate per 1,000 person-years was 2.10 from CHD events and 3.78 from non-CHD causes.

The behavior pattern was classified at intake from the tape-recorded, structured interview developed for this purpose (Rosenman, et al. 1964) and administered by trained interviewers. The final rating was made after audition of the tape-recorded interview and without knowledge of other intake-history or measurement. This was done to avoid possible bias introduced by knowledge of subjects' other attributes. The 3,154 subjects at risk included 1,589 assessed as exhibiting type A behavior patterns and 1,565 assessed as exhibiting type B behavior patterns. Death from CHD events occurred in thirty-four type A and sixteen type B subjects and from non-CHD causes in fifty-one type A and thirty-nine type B subjects, including five type A and two type B subjects with manifest CHD. The death rate per 1,000 person-years was 2.92 for type A and 1.32 for type B subjects for CHD causes, and 4.38 for type A and 3.21 for type B subjects for non-CHD causes. The 2,391 subjects without manifest CHD included 1,129 type A and 1,262 type B subjects. The 506 men who were lost on or before final follow-up are also considered to be non-CHD cases and include 282 type A and 224 type B subjects. The total number of person-years of follow-up was 11,642 for type A and 12,148 for type B subjects. Thus, there was a slightly greater loss to follow-up of type A than of type B men, pro-portionately speaking. The excess of type A men in the CHD incidence group, accordingly, is not a function of a greater loss of type B subjects from the initial populations at risk. Association between behavior pattern and CHD is slightly underestimated by using CHD rates based on number at risk at intake rather than on person-years of exposure to risk. Nevertheless, in what follows, rates based on number at risk at intake are required by the multivariate adjustment method, to be described here, that plays a major role in data analysis.

All electrocardiograms were screened by a cardiologist while those considered definitely or probably indicative of myocardial infarction were referred to an independent medical referee who was solely responsible for all diagnosis of manifest CHD, and this selection was made in the absence of any knowledge of the variables under investigation (Rosenman, *et al.* 1964).

The category termed 'symptomatic myocardial infarction (MI)' includes 135 subjects, of whom thirty-one died in association with their initial CHD event. The diagnosis of acute MI in 104 surviving subjects was based on the occurrence of a symptomatic CHD event accompanied by definitive electrocardiographic and serum enzyme changes. Post-mortem examination was performed on twenty-four of the thirty-one deceased subjects and demonstrated the presence of acute coronary thrombosis or acute MI in twenty-three instances and of severe, diffuse, coronary atherosclerosis in one subject, who was found dead in bed. No other anatomic or toxicological findings were noted to controvert inclusion of this subject as a case of sudden CHD death. The diagnosis of acute MI was confirmed by ante-mortem hospital findings in four of the seven deceased subjects who were not autopsied. Three other deceased subjects who were not autopsied were included because of sudden death (one subject died suddenly while driving his car). None of the three had any other acute or chronic illness that might controvert including them as cases of sudden CHD death.

The category termed 'unrecognized MI' is herein used to designate seventy-one subjects whose interval ECG during annual resurvey was adjudged by the independent electrocardiographer and medical referee to show definite evidence of the occurrence of MI that, however, was either 'silent' or clinically unrecognized. The category of 'angina pectoris (without MI)' was devised for fifty-one subjects by the medical referee, on the basis of the development of classical Heberden disease, and excluded subjects whose symptoms were atypical or doubtful.

The analyses are based on intake data, except for fasting serum triglyceride levels, which were determined at the first annual resurvey examination. Among the 578 subjects with a history of parental CHD, 481 (83.2 per cent) reported it at intake and the remaining ninety-seven (16.8 per cent) reported this during the first five years of follow-up. The statistical significance of categorical data was analyzed by the χ^2 test, and of continuous variables by student t-test. For behaviour pattern, a multivariate adjustment using the Mantel–Haenszel χ^2 method of analysis was utilized (Mantel and Haenszel 1959). The association between behaviour pattern and CHD incidence was adjusted one at a time and then in combination with other risk factors that were associated with the behavior pattern.

Results

Single predictive factors and CHD incidence

There were 3,154 intake subjects at risk for initial occurrence of CHD, 2,249 of whom were aged thirty-nine to forty-nine years, and 905 aged fifty to fifty-nine years. Clinical CHD was observed in 257 subjects during the mean eight and a half years of follow-up, an average annual incidence of 9.6/1,000 subjects at risk.

The educational level was inversely related to CHD incidence in both age groups, although annual income was not related to CHD rates. Subjects with a history of parental CHD and those with reported diabetes each exhibited higher CHD incidence of about the same proportion in both age groups, but statistical significance was not reached in the older group because of the small number of subjects. This exemplifies the difficulty in interpreting the possible difference between clinical and statistical significance. For example, the rate of CHD in older subjects with parental history of CHD was 5.4 per cent higher than in those without such history while the corresponding increment in the younger group was only 4 per cent. Nevertheless, because of the respective differences in the numbers of subjects involved, the observed findings reached statistical significance only in the younger group. However, the magnitude of the observed differences suggests clinical significance in both age groups.

Reported occupational-physical activity was not associated with differences in CHD rates. However, men reporting regular exercise habits (daily, purposeful calisthenics, walking, or hobby exercise) had lower CHD rates than those reporting only occasional avocational exercise, and differences were significant in the older group. Smoking habits were related to CHD incidence in both decades – with higher rates for current cigarette smokers – and rates of CHD were significantly related to reported daily amount smoked at intake.

There was no significant difference in the average weight gain between age twenty-five years and intake for subjects with or without CHD. However, subjects suffering CHD exhibited higher mean weights at intake. Average systolic and diastolic blood pressures, and serum levels of cholesterol and triglycerides, and beta-alpha-lipoprotein ratios were significantly higher in subjects of both age groups who later had CHD, compared to the non-CHD population, and the CHD rate was proportional to the degree of measured level of each factor. Significantly higher rates of CHD were observed in subjects of both age groups classified at intake as type A compared to those with the type B behavior pattern.

CHD incidence and behavior pattern
In view of the association of type A with other risk factors for CHD, it was important to re-examine the incidence of CHD in type A and type B subjects stratified against all factors found to be significantly related to the CHD incidence (Rosenman, *et al.* 1970). The results of this survey are shown in *Table 36* (see over). The higher CHD incidence in type A subjects prevailed when subjects were stratified by each of the predictive risk factors. The type A and type B subjects exhibited no significant differences of mean age, height, or weight. These results were corrected for each single risk factor in studying the association between the behavior pattern and the CHD incidence. No single risk factor had a substantial impact on the degree of association.

The possibility that the combination of effects of all risk factors may explain a substantial part of the behavior pattern-CHD association than was studied by the Mantel–Haenszel procedure (Mantel and Haenszel 1959) in each age group. This method of analysis, in addition to providing a test of statistical significance, gives a summary measure of association, which is computed in a way that is analogous to direct adjustment of rates. The resulting measure can be interpreted, in this case, as an approximate relative risk that gives the ratio of the CHD rate in type A subjects divided by the CHD rate in type B subjects.

In this analysis, the behavior pattern-CHD relationship was viewed when simultaneous adjustment was made for parental history of CHD, current cigarette usage, systolic and diastolic blood pressure, serum levels of cholesterol and triglyceride, and beta-alpha-lipoprotein ratios, all treated as categorical variables as indicated in *Table 36*. Simultaneous adjustment eliminates any apparent increase of CHD risk in type A subjects that stems from the tendency of these subjects to have a relatively higher occurrence of any of these other risk factors. In the younger age group, the approximate relative risk – odds ratio (Fleiss 1973) – which assesses the association between behavior pattern and CHD incidence is 2.21 ($P < .0001$) before adjustment and 1.87 ($P < .003$) after adjustment for the other risk factors. In the older group, the ratio is 2.31 ($P < .0002$) before adjustment and 1.98 ($P < .019$) after adjustment. The results of these analyses thus indicated that the predictive relationship of the behavior pattern to the CHD incidence could not be 'explained away' by other risk factors, a finding similar to that at the four and a half-year follow-up in which the same issue was studied

Table 36   *Prospective history and findings by behavior pattern*

| | age 39–49 yr | | | | | | age 50–59 yr | | | | | |
| | subjects at risk | | subjects with CHD* | | rate of CHD† | | subjects at risk | | subjects with CHD | | rate of CHD† | |
	type A	type B	type A	type B	type A	type B	type A	type B	type A	type B	type A	type B
no. of subjects	1,067	1,182	95	50	10.5	5.0	522	383	83	29	18.7	8.9
parental history of CHD												
yes	214	197	23	15	12.6	9.0	103	64	20	7	22.8	12.9
no	853	985	72	35	9.9	4.2	419	319	63	22	17.7	8.1
smoking habits												
never smoked	221	315	11	8	5.9	3.0	90	89	10	5	13.1	6.6
pipe or cigar	191	216	11	6	6.8	3.3	81	78	17	2	24.7	3.0
former cigarette	110	129	11	5	11.8	4.6	91	41	10	2	12.9	5.7
current cigarette	545	522	62	31	13.4	7.0	260	175	46	20	20.8	13.4
current cigarette usage												
none	522	660	33	19	7.4	3.4	262	208	37	9	16.6	5.1
1–15 day	95	119	3	8	3.7	7.9	65	43	8	1	14.5	2.7
≥16 day	450	403	59	23	15.4	11.4	195	132	38	19	22.9	16.9
systolic blood pressure, mm Hg												
<120	264	328	17	4	7.6	1.4	95	80	7	4	8.7	5.9
120–159	771	826	69	43	10.5	6.1	381	283	64	21	19.8	8.7
≥160	32	28	9	3	33.1	12.6	46	20	12	4	30.7	23.5

diastolic blood pressure, mm Hg												
<95	970	1,100	81	45	9.8	4.8	448	344	64	25	16.8	8.5
≥95	97	82	14	5	17.0	7.2	74	39	19	4	30.2	12.1
serum cholesterol, mg/100 ml												
<220	486	607	24	11	5.8	2.1	211	148	20	6	11.2	4.8
220–259	352	376	32	20	10.7	6.3	179	142	36	10	23.7	8.3
≥260	226	195	39	19	20.3	11.5	130	90	27	13	24.4	17.0
fasting serum triglycerides, mg/100 ml												
<100	−252	348	−12	7	5.6	2.4	151	99	16	5	12.5	5.9
100–176	500	538	48	22	11.3	4.8	238	170	37	11	18.3	7.6
≥177	247	249	30	20	14.3	9.6	114	98	26	9	26.8	10.8
serum β-/α-lipoprotein ratio												
<2.36	733	836	57	24	9.1	3.4	323	263	43	18	15.7	8.1
≥2.36	331	343	38	26	13.5	8.9	196	117	39	11	23.4	11.1

* coronary heart disease

† average annual rate/1,000 subjects at risk. Difference of rates between type A and type B subjects are tested for significance by Mantel–Haenszel χ^2, with adjustment for factors indicated. For each factor the adjusted association between behavior pattern and CHD incidence is significant at $P < .001$.

by means of both bivariate and multivariate analyses (Rosenman, *et al.* 1970).

Comment

Epidemiological studies have confirmed a relationship between the incidence of clinical CHD and prospective risk factors, including age, parental history of premature CHD, elevated systolic and diastolic blood pressures, cigarette smoking, and higher serum concentrations of cholesterol, triglycerides, and beta-alpha-lipoproteins. These findings are again confirmed in the present eight and a half-year follow-up of a large population. However, the predictive relationship of any single risk factor with the incidence of CHD may be a reflection of its association with other risk factors. Accordingly, any attempts at causal interpretation of the data observed in these univariate analyses requires caution. It is beyond the scope of the present report to investigate the multivariate relationships of all of the risk factors studied herein, as was done for the behavior pattern. Although these factors are important in prediction of relative risk of CHD, even the combination of such risk factors cannot definitively predict CHD in prospective studies of middle-aged American men, indicating that other variables must play an important pathogenetic role in the CHD incidence (Keys 1972).

The present findings reaffirm earlier follow-up studies (Rosenman, *et al.* 1970) and indicate that the overt behavior pattern is prominent among variables in the list of major risk factors. The results also confirm that this relationship is not the artifact of the association of the behavior pattern with other risk factors and suggest that the pathogenetic force of type A behavior on the CHD incidence is due primarily to factors other than the classical risk factors, perhaps operating through various neurohormonal pathways. However, it seems clear that behavior pattern A indicates a pathogenetic force operating in addition to, as well as in conjunction with, the classical risk factors.

The findings would appear to have important clinical implications for the primary prevention of CHD. Moreover, evaluating patients with CHD for presence of the coronary-prone behavior pattern may well improve the prognostic prediction of the course of the disease. It has not yet been shown whether altering facets of the behavior pattern in surviving type A CHD patients reduce their risk of reinfarction, but research along these lines is strongly indicated.

PART IX
The social definition of illness

27 Decision rules, types of error, and their consequences in medical diagnosis

*Thomas J. Scheff**

[This paper has been edited from the original according to the editors' general strategy with the presentation of an algebraic equation for the assessment of the costs and benefits of medical treatment being completely deleted. The author is Professor of Sociology in the USA.]

The purpose of this paper is to describe one important norm for handling uncertainty in medical diagnosis, that judging a sick person well is more to be avoided than judging a well person sick, and to suggest some of the consequences of the application of this norm in medical practice. Apparently this norm, like many important cultural norms, 'goes without saying' in the sub-culture of the medical profession; in form, however, it resembles any decision rule for guiding behavior under conditions of uncertainty. In the discussion that follows, decision rules in law, statistics, and medicine are compared, in order to indicate the types of error that are thought to be the more important to avoid and the assumptions underlying this preference. On the basis of recent findings of the widespread distribution of elements of disease and deviance in normal populations, the assumption of a uniform relationship between disease signs and impairment is criticized. Finally, it is

* extracted from *Behavioural Science* (1963) 8 (2): 97–107, April

suggested that to the extent that physicians are guided by this medical decision rule, they too often place patients in the 'sick role' who could otherwise have continued in their normal pursuits.

Decision rules

To the extent that physicians and the public are biased towards treatment, the 'creation' of illness, i.e., the production of unnecessary impairment, may go hand in hand with the prevention and treatment of disease in modern medicine. The magnitude of the bias towards treatment in any single case may be quite small, since there are probably other medical decision rules ('When in doubt, delay your decision') which counteract the rule discussed here. Even a small bias, however, if it is relatively constant throughout Western society, can have effects of large magnitude. Since this argument is based largely on fragmentary evidence, it is intended merely to stimulate further discussion and research, rather than to demonstrate the validity of a point of view. The discussion will begin with the consideration of a decision rule in law.

In criminal trials in England and the United States, there is an explicit rule for arriving at decisions in the face of uncertainty: 'A man is innocent until proven guilty.' The meaning of this rule is made clear by the English common law definition of the phrase 'proven guilty', which according to tradition is that the judge or jury must find the evidence of guilt compelling *beyond a reasonable doubt*. The basic legal rule for arriving at a decision in the face of uncertainty may be briefly stated: 'When in doubt, acquit.' That is, the jury or judge must not be equally wary of erroneously convicting or acquitting: the error that is most important to avoid is to erroneously convict. This concept is expressed in the maxim, 'Better a thousand guilty men go free, than one innocent man be convicted'.

The reasons underlying this rule seem clear. It is assumed that in most cases, a conviction will do irreversible harm to an individual by damaging his reputation in the eyes of his fellows. The individual is seen as weak and defenseless, relative to society, and therefore in no position to sustain the consequences of an erroneous decision. An erroneous acquittal, on the other hand, damages society. If an individual who has actually committed a crime is not punished, he may commit the crime again, or more important, the deterrent effect of punishment for the violation of this crime may be diminished for others. Although these are serious outcomes they are generally thought not to be as serious as the consequences of erroneous conviction for the innocent individual, since society is able to sustain an indefinite number of such errors without serious consequences. For these and perhaps other reasons, the decision rule to assume innocence exerts a powerful influence on legal proceedings.

Type 1 and type 2 errors

Decision on guilt or innocence is a special case of a problem to which statisticians have given considerable attention, the testing of hypotheses. Since most scientific work is done with samples, statisticians have developed techniques to guard against results which are due to chance sampling fluctuations. The problem, however, is that one might reject a finding as due to sampling fluctuations which was actually correct. There are, therefore, two kinds of errors: rejecting a hypothesis which is true, and accepting one which is false. Usually the hypothesis is stated so that the former error (rejecting a hypothesis which is true) is the error that is thought to be the more important to avoid. This kind of error is called an 'error of the first kind', or a type 1 error. The latter error (accepting a hypothesis which is false) is the less important error to avoid, and is called an 'error of the second kind', or a type 2 error (Neyman 1950: 265–66).

To guard against chance fluctuations in sampling, statisticians test the probability that findings could have arisen by chance. At some predetermined probability (called the alpha level) usually 0.5 or less, the possibility that the findings arose by chance is rejected. This level means that there are five chances in a hundred that one will reject a hypothesis which is true. Although these five chances indicate a real risk of error, it is not common to set the level much lower (say .001) because this raises the probability of making an error of the second kind.

Although the legal decision rule is not expressed in as precise a form as a statistical decision rule, it represents a very similar procedure for dealing with uncertainty. There is one respect, however, in which it is quite different. Statistical decision procedures are recognized by those who use them as mere conveniences, which can be varied according to the circumstances. The legal decision rule, in contrast, is an inflexible and binding moral rule, which carries with it the force of long sanction and tradition. The assumption of innocence is a part of the social institution of law in Western society; it is explicitly stated in legal codes, and is accepted as legitimate by jurists and usually by the general populace, with only occasional grumbling, e.g., a criminal is seen as 'getting off' because of 'legal technicalities'.

Decision rules in medicine

Although the analogous rule for decisions in medicine is not as explicitly stated as the rule in law and probably is considerably less rigid, it would seem that there is such a rule in medicine which is as imperative in its operation as its analogue in law. Do physicians and the general public consider that rejecting the hypothesis of illness when it is true, or accepting it when it is false, is the error that is most important to avoid? It seems fairly clear that the rule in medicine may be stated as: 'When in doubt, continue to suspect illness.' That is, for a physician to dismiss a patient when he is actually ill is a type 1 error, and to retain a patient when he is not ill is a type 2 error.

Most physicians learn early in their training that it is far more culpable to dismiss a sick patient than to retain a well one. This rule is so pervasive and fundamental that it goes unstated in textbooks on diagnosis. It is occasionally mentioned explicitly in other contexts, however. Neyman, for example, in his discussion of X-ray screening for tuberculosis, states:

> '[If the patient is actually well, but the hypothesis that he is sick is accepted, [a Type 2 error] then the patient will suffer some unjustified anxiety and, perhaps, will be put to some unnecessary expense until further studies of his health will establish that any alarm about the state of his chest is unfounded. Also, the unjustified precautions ordered by the clinic may somewhat affect its reputation. On the other hand, should the hypothesis [of sickness] be true and if the accepted hypothesis be [that he is well, a Type 1 error], then the patient will be in danger of losing the precious opportunity of treating the incipient disease in its beginning stages when the cure is not so difficult. Furthermore, the oversight by the clinic's specialist of the dangerous condition would affect the clinic's reputation even more than the unnecessary alarm. From this point of view, it appears that the error of rejecting the hypothesis [of sickness] when it is true is *far more important* to avoid than the error of accepting the hypothesis [of illness] when it is false.]' (Neyman 1950: 270, italics added)

Although this particular discussion pertains to tuberculosis it is pertinent to many other diseases also. From casual conversations with physicians, the impression one gains is that this moral lesson is deeply ingrained in the physician's personal code.

It is not only physicians who feel this way, however. This rule is grounded both in legal proceedings and in popular sentiment. Although there is some sentiment against type 2 errors (unnecessary surgery, for instance), it has nothing like the force and urgency of the sentiment against type 1 errors. A physician who dismisses a patient who subsequently dies of a disease that should have been detected is not only subject to legal action for negligence and possible loss of license for incompetence, but also to moral condemnation from his colleagues and from his own conscience for his delinquency. Nothing remotely resembling this amount of moral and legal suasion is brought to bear for committing a type 2 error. Indeed, this error is sometimes seen as sound clinical practice, indicating a healthily conservative approach to medicine.

The discussion to this point suggests that physicians follow a decision rule which may be stated, 'When in doubt, diagnose illness'. If physicians are actually influenced by this rule, then studies of the validity of diagnosis should demonstrate the operation of the rule. That is, we should expect that objective studies of diagnostic errors should show that type 1 and type 2 errors do not occur with equal frequency, but in fact, that type 2 errors far outnumber type 1 errors. Unfortunately for our purposes, however, there are apparently only a few studies which provide the type of data which would adequately test the hypothesis. Although studies of the reliability of diagnosis abound (Garland 1959), showing that physicians disagree with each other in their diagnoses of the same patients, these studies do not report the validity of diagnosis, or the types of error which are made, with the following exceptions: we can infer that type 2 errors outnumber type 1 errors from Bakwin's study of physicians' judgments regarding the advisability of tonsillectomy for 1,000 schoolchildren.

> 'Of these, some 611 had had their tonsils removed. The remaining 389 were then examined by other physicians, and 174 were selected for tonsillectomy. This left 215 children whose tonsils were apparently normal. Another group of doctors was put to work examining these 215 children, and 99 of them were adjudged in need of tonsillectomy. Still another group of doctors was then employed to examine the remaining children, and nearly one-half were recommended for operation.' (Bakwin 1945: 693)

Almost half of each group of children was adjudged to be in need of the operation. Even assuming that a small proportion of children needing tonsillectomy were missed in each examination (type 1 error), the number of type 2 errors in this study far exceeded the number of type 1 errors.

In the field of roentgenology, studies of diagnostic error are apparently more highly developed than in other areas of medicine. Garland (1959:

31) summarizes these findings, reporting that in a study of 14,867 films for tuberculosis signs, there were 1,216 positive readings which turned out to be clinically negative (type 2 error) and only twenty-four negative readings which turned out to be clinically active (type 1 error)! This ratio is apparently a fairly typical finding in roentgenographic studies. Since physicians are well aware of the provisional nature of radiological findings, this great discrepancy between the frequency of types of error in film screening is not too alarming. On the other hand, it does provide objective evidence of the operation of the decision rule 'Better safe than sorry'.

The logic of this (better safe than sorry) decision rule rests on two assumptions:

1 Disease is usually a determinate, inevitably unfolding process, which, if undetected and untreated, will grow to a point where it endangers the life or limb of the individual, and in the case of contagious diseases, the lives of others. This is not to say, of course, that physicians think of all diseases as determinate: witness the concept of the 'benign' condition. The point here is that the imagery of disease which the physician uses in attempting to reach a decision, his working hypothesis, is *usually* based on the deterministic model of disease.

2 Medical diagnosis of illness, unlike legal judgment, is not an irreversible act which does untold damage to the status and reputation of the patient. A physician may search for illness for an indefinitely long time, causing inconvenience for the patient, perhaps, but in the typical case doing the patient no irradicable harm. Obviously, again, physicians do not *always* make this assumption. A physician who suspects epilepsy in a truck driver knows full well that his patient will probably never drive a truck again if the diagnosis is made, and the physician will go to great lengths to avoid a type 2 error in this situation. Similarly, if a physician suspects that a particular patient has hypochondriacal trends, the physician will lean in the direction of a type 1 error in a situation of uncertainty. These and other similar situations are exceptions, however. The physician's *usual* working assumption is that medical observation and diagnosis, in itself, is neutral and innocuous, relative to the dangers resulting from disease.

In the light of these two assumptions, therefore, it is seen as far better for the physician to chance a type 2 error than a type 1 error. These two assumptions will be examined and criticized in the remainder of the paper. The assumption that type 2 errors are relatively harmless will be considered first.

In recent discussions it is increasingly recognized that in one area of medicine, psychiatry, the assumption that medical diagnosis can cause no irreversible harm to the patient's status is dubious. Psychiatric treatment, in many segments of the population and for many occupations, raises a question about the person's social status. It could be argued that in making a medical diagnosis the psychiatrist comes very close to making a legal decision, with its ensuing consequences for the person's reputation. One might argue that the type 2 error in psychiatry, of judging a well person sick, is at least as much to be avoided as the type 1 error, of judging the sick person well. Yet the psychiatrist's moral orientation, since he is first and foremost a physician, is guided by the medical, rather than the legal decision rule. The psychiatrist continues to be more willing to err on the conservative side, to diagnose as ill when the person is healthy, even though it is no longer clear that this error is any more desirable than its opposite.

There is a more fundamental question about this decision rule, however, which concerns both physical illness and mental disorder. This question primarily concerns the first assumption, that disease is a determinate process. It also implicates the second assumption, that medical treatment does not have irreversible effects.

A consideration of disease signs and deviant behavior among psychiatric patients suggests that in order to know the probability that a person with a disease sign would become incapacitated because of the development of disease, investigations quite unlike existing studies would need to be conducted. These would be longitudinal studies of outcomes in persons having signs of disease in a random sample of a normal population, in which no attempt was made to arrest the disease. It is true that there are a number of longitudinal studies in which the effects of treatment are compared with the effects of non-treatment. These studies, however, have usually been conducted with clinical groups, rather than with persons with disease signs who were located in field studies. Even clinical trials appear to offer many difficulties, both from the ethical and scientific points of view (Hill 1960). These difficulties would be increased many times in controlled field trials, as would the problems which concern the amount of time and money necessary. Without such studies, nevertheless, the meaning of many common disease signs remains somewhat equivocal.

If, as has been argued here, such illness goes unattended without serious consequences, the assumption that medical diagnosis has no irreversible effects on the patient seems questionable. The patient's attitude to his illness is usually considerably changed during and by the series of physical examinations. These changes, which may profoundly influence the course of a chronic illness, are not taken seriously by the medical profession and, though occasionally mentioned, they have never been the subject of a proper scientific investigation (Balint 1957: 43).

There are grounds for believing that persons who avail themselves of professional services are under considerable strain and tension (if the problem could have been easily solved, they would probably have used more informal means of handling it). Social-psychological principles indicate that persons under strain are highly suggestible, particularly to suggestions from a prestigious source, such as a physician.

It can be argued that the type 2 error involves the danger of having a person enter the 'sick role' (Parsons 1950) in circumstances where no serious result would ensue if the illness were unattended. Perhaps the combination of a physician determined to find disease *signs*, if they are to be found, and the suggestible patient, searching for subjective *symptoms* among the many amorphous and usually unattended bodily impulses, is often sufficient to unearth a disease which changes the patient's status from that of well to sick, and may also have effects on his familial and occupational status. (In Lemert's terms (1951), the illness would be *secondary deviation* after the person has entered the sick role.)

There is a considerable body of evidence in the medical literature concerning the process in which the physician unnecessarily causes the patient to enter the sick role. Thus, in a discussion of 'iatrogenic' (physician-induced heart disease) this point is made:

> 'The physician, by calling attention to a murmur or some cardiovascular abnormality, even though functionally insignificant, may precipitate [symptoms of heart disease]. The experience of the work classification units of cardiac-in-industry programs, where patients with cardiovascular disease are evaluated as to work capacity, gives impressive evidence regarding the high incidence of such functional manifestations in persons with the diagnosis of cardiac lesion.'
> (Warren & Wolter 1954: 78)

Although there is a tendency in medicine to dismiss this process as due to quirks of particular patients, e.g., as malingering, hypochondriasis, or as 'merely functional disease' (that is, functional for the patient), causation probably lies not in the patient, but in medical procedures. Most people, perhaps, if they actually have the disease signs and are told by an authority, the physician, that they are ill, will obligingly come up with appropriate symptoms.

Implications for research

The hypothesis suggested by the preceding discussion is that physicians and the public typically overvalue medical treatment relative to non-treatment as a course of action in the face of uncertainty, and that this overvaluation results in the creation as well as the prevention of impairment. This hypothesis, since it is based on scattered observations, is put forward only to point out several areas where systematic research is needed.

From the point of view of assessing the effectiveness of medical practice, this hypothesis is probably too general to be used directly. Needed for such a task are hypotheses concerning the conditions under which error is likely to occur, the type of error that is likely, and the consequences of each type of error. Significant dimensions of the amount and type of error and its consequences would appear to be characteristics of the disease, the physician, the patient, and the organizational setting in which diagnosis takes place.

To the extent that future research can indicate the conditions which influence the amount, type, and consequences of error, such research can make direct contributions to medical practice. Two types of research seem necessary. First, in order to establish the true risks of impairment associated with common disease signs, controlled field trials of treated and untreated outcomes in a normal population would be needed. Second, perhaps in conjunction with these field trials, experimental studies of the effect of suggestion of illness by physicians and others would be necessary to determine the risks of unnecessary entry into the sick role.

28 Medicine as an institution of social control: the medicalizing of society

*Irving Kenneth Zola**

[*This paper has been edited from the original by reducing the number of examples and by deleting a lengthy historical discussion of the changing role of medicine in society in which the author demonstrates the close relationship between medical activity and moral judgement. The author is Professor of Sociology in the USA.*]

The theme of this essay is that medicine is becoming a major institution of social control, nudging aside, if not incorporating, the more traditional institutions of religion and law. It is becoming the new repository of truth, the place where absolute and often final judgements are made by supposedly morally neutral and objective experts. And these judgements are made, not in the name of virtue or legitimacy, but in the name of health. Moreover, this is not occurring through the political power physicians hold or can influence, but is largely an insidious and often undramatic phenomenon accomplished by 'medicalizing' much of daily living, by making medicine and the labels 'healthy' and 'ill' *relevant* to an ever increasing part of human existence.

The full exercise of medical influence is, however, a twentieth-century phenomenon. Only now is the process of 'medicalization' upon us – a phenomenon which Freidson has operationalized most succinctly. 'The medical profession has first claim to jurisdiction over the label of illness

* extracted from the *Sociological Review* (1972) **20** (4): 487–504, new series

and anything to which it may be attached, irrespective of its capacity to deal with it effectively' (Freidson 1970: 251). For illustrative purposes this 'attaching' process may be categorized in four concrete ways: first, through the expansion of what in life is deemed relevant to the good practice of medicine; second, through the retention of absolute control over certain technical procedures; third, through the retention of near absolute access to certain 'taboo' areas; and finally, through the expansion of what in medicine is deemed relevant to the good practice of life.

The expansion of what in life is deemed relevant to the good practice of medicine

The change of medicine's commitment from a specific aetiological model of disease to a multi-causal one and the greater acceptance of the concepts of comprehensive medicine, psychosomatics, etc, have enormously expanded that which is or can be relevant to the understanding, treatment, and even prevention of disease. Thus it is no longer necessary for the patient merely to divulge the symptoms of his body, but also the symptoms of daily living, his habits and his worries.

It is not merely, however, the nature of the data needed to make more accurate diagnoses and treatments, but the perspective which accompanies it – a perspective which pushes the physician far beyond his office and the exercise of technical skills. To rehabilitate or at least alleviate many of the ravages of chronic disease, it has become increasingly necessary to intervene to change permanently the habits of a patient's lifetime – be it of working, sleeping, playing, or eating. In prevention the 'extension into life' becomes even deeper, since the very idea of primary prevention means getting there *before* the disease process starts. The physician must not only seek out his clientele but once found must often convince them that they must do something *now* and perhaps at a time when the potential patient feels well or not especially troubled. If this in itself does not get the prevention-oriented physician involved in the workings of society, then the nature of 'effective' mechanisms for intervention surely does, as illustrated by the statement of a physician trying to deal with health problems in the ghetto: 'Any effort to improve the health of ghetto residents cannot be separated from equal and simultaneous efforts to remove the multiple social, political and economic restraints currently imposed on inner city residents' (Norman 1969).

Certain forms of social intervention and control emerge even when medicine comes to grips with some of its more traditional problems like heart disease and cancer. An increasing number of physicians feel that a change in diet may be the most effective deterrent to a number of cardiovascular complications. They are, however, so perplexed as to how to get the general population to follow their recommendations that a leading article in a national magazine was entitled 'To Save the Heart: Diet by Decree?' (*Time*: 1968: 42). And what will be the implications of even stronger evidence which links age at parity, frequency of sexual intercourse, or the lack of male circumcision to the incidence of cervical cancer, can be left to our imagination!

Through the retention of absolute control over certain technical procedures

In particular this refers to skills which in certain jurisdictions are the very operational and legal definition of the practice of medicine – the right to do surgery and prescribe drugs. Both of these take medicine far beyond concern with ordinary organic disease.

In surgery this is seen in several different sub-specialities. The plastic surgeon has at least participated in, if not helped perpetuate, certain aesthetic standards. What once was a practice confined to restoration has now expanded beyond the correction of certain traumatic or even congenital deformities to the creation of new physical properties, from size of nose to size of breast, as well as dealing with certain phenomena – wrinkles, sagging, etc – formerly associated with the 'natural' process of ageing. Alterations in sexual and reproductive functioning have long been a medical concern. Yet today the frequency of hysterectomies seems not so highly correlated as one might think with the presence of organic disease. (What avenues the very possibility of sex change will open is anyone's guess.) Transplantations, despite their still relative infrequency, have had a tremendous effect on our very notions of death and dying. And at the other end of life's continuum, since abortion is still essentially a surgical procedure, it is to the physician–surgeon that society is turning (and the physician–surgeon accepting) for criteria and guidelines.

In the exclusive right to prescribe and thus pronounce on and regulate drugs, the power of the physician is even more awesome. Forgetting for the moment our obsession with youth's 'illegal' use of drugs, any observer can see, judging by sales alone, that the greatest increase in drug use over the last ten years has not been in the realm of treating any organic disease but in treating a large number of psycho-social states. Thus we have drugs for nearly every mood: to help us sleep or keep us awake; to enhance our appetite or decrease it; to tone down our energy level or to increase it; to relieve our depression or stimulate our interest.

Through the retention of near absolute access to certain 'taboo' areas

These 'taboo' areas refer to medicine's almost exclusive licence to examine and treat that most personal of individual possessions – the inner workings of our bodies and minds. My contention is that if anything can be shown in some way to affect the workings of the body and to a lesser extent the mind, then it can be labelled an 'illness' itself or jurisdictionally 'a medical problem'. In a sheer statistical sense the import of this is especially great if we look at only four such problems – ageing, drug addiction, alcoholism, and pregnancy. The first and last were once regarded as normal natural processes and the middle two as human foibles and weaknesses. Now this has changed and to some extent medical specialities have emerged to meet these new needs. Numerically this expands medicine's involvement not only in a longer span of human existence, but it opens the possibility of medicine's services to millions if not billions of people.

Through the expansion of what in medicine is deemed relevant to the good practice of life

Though in some ways this is the most powerful of all the 'medicalizing of society' processes, the point can be made simply. Here we refer to the use of medical rhetoric and evidence in the arguments to advance any cause. To paraphrase Wootton (Wootton 1959) today the prestige of *any* proposal is immensely enhanced, if not justified, when it is expressed in the idiom of medical science. To say that many who use such labels are not professionals only begs the issue, for the public is only taking its cues from professionals who increasingly have been extending their expertise into the social sphere or have called for such an extension (Alinsky 1967; Wedge 1961). In politics one hears of the healthy or unhealthy economy or state. More concretely, the physical and mental health of American presidential candidates has been an issue in the last four elections and a recent book claimed to link faulty political decisions with faulty health (L'Etang 1970). For years we knew that the environment was unattractive, polluted, noisy, and, in certain ways, dying, but now we learn that its death may not be unrelated to our own demise. To end with a rather mundane if depressing example, there has always been a constant battle between school authorities and their charges on the basis of dress and such habits as smoking, but recently the issue was happily resolved for a local school administration when they declared that such restrictions were necessary for reasons of health.

The potential and consequences of medical control

The list of daily activities to which health can be related is ever growing and with the current operating perspective of medicine it seems infinitely expandable. The reasons are manifold. It is not merely that medicine has extended its jurisdiction to cover new problems (Szasz 1961; Leifer 1969) or that doctors are professionally committed to finding disease (Freidson 1970; Scheff 1964) nor even that society keeps creating disease (Dubos 1959; Dubos 1965). For if none of these obtained today we should still find medicine exerting an enormous influence on society. The most powerful empirical stimulus for this is the realization of how much everyone has or believes he has something organically wrong with him, or put more positively, how much can be done to make one feel, look, or function better.

The rates of 'clinical entities' found on surveys or by periodic health examinations range upwards from 50 to 80 per cent of the population studied (Meigs 1961; Siegel 1963). We used to rationalize that this high level of prevalence did not, however, translate itself into action since not only are rates of medical utilization not astonishingly high but they also have not gone up appreciably. Some recent studies, however, indicate that we may have been looking in the wrong place for this medical action. It has been noted in the United States and the United Kingdom that within a given twenty-four to thirty-six hour period, from 50 to 80 per cent of the adult population have taken one or more 'medical' drugs (Dunnell and Cartwright 1972; White, *et al.* 1967).

The belief in the omnipresence of disorder is further enhanced by a reading of the scientific, pharmacological, and medical literature, for there one finds a growing litany of indictments of 'unhealthy' life activities. From sex to food, from aspirins to clothes, from driving your car to riding the surf, it seems that under certain conditions, or in combination with certain other substances or activities or if done too much or too little, virtually anything can lead to certain medical problems. In short, I at least have finally been convinced that living in injurious to health. This remark is not meant as facetiously as it may sound. But rather every aspect of our daily life has in it elements of risk to health.

These facts take on particular importance not only when health becomes a paramount value in society, but also a phenomenon whose diagnosis and treatment have been restricted to a certain group. For this means that that group, perhaps unwittingly, is in a position to exercise great control and influence about what we should and should not do to attain that 'paramount value'.

Freidson (1970) has very cogently analyzed why the expert in general and the medical expert in particular should be granted a certain autonomy in his researches, his diagnosis, and his recommended treatments. On the other hand, when it comes to constraining or directing human behaviour *because* of the data of his researches, diagnosis, and treatment, a different situation obtains. For in these kinds of decisions it seems that too often the physician is guided not by his technical knowledge but by his values, or values latent in his very techniques.

It would seem that the value positions of those on both sides of the abortion issue need little documenting, but let us pause briefly at a field where 'harder' scientists are at work – genetics. The issue of genetic counselling, or whether life should be allowed to begin at all, can only be an ever increasing one. As we learn more and more about congenital, inherited disorders or predispositions, and as the population size for whatever reason becomes more limited, then inevitably there will follow an attempt to improve the quality of the population which shall be produced. At a conference on the more limited concern of what to do when there is a documented probability of the offspring of certain unions being damaged, a position was taken that it was not necessary to pass laws or bar marriages that might produce such offspring. Recognizing the power and influence of medicine and the doctor, one of those present argued: 'There is no reason why sensible people could not be dissuaded from marrying if they know that one out of four of their children is likely to inherit a disease' (Eisenberg 1966). There are in this statement certain values on marriage and what it is or could be that, while they may be popular, are not necessarily shared by all. Thus, in addition to presenting the argument against marriage, it would seem that the doctor should – if he were to engage in the issue at all – present at the same time some of the other alternatives:

> Some 'parents' could be willing to live with the risk that out of four children, three may turn out fine. Depending on the diagnostic procedures available they could take the risk and if indications were negative abort.
> If this risk were too great but the desire to bear children was there, and depending on the type of problem, artificial insemination might be a possibility. Barring all these and not wanting to take any risk, they could adopt children.
> Finally, there is the option of being married without having any children.

Conclusion

C. S. Lewis warned more than a quarter of a century ago that 'man's power over Nature is really the power of some men over other men, with Nature as their instrument'. The same could be said regarding man's power over health and illness. For the labels health and illness are remarkable 'depoliticizers' of an issue. By locating the source and the treatment of problems in an individual, other levels of intervention are effectively closed. By the very acceptance of a specific behaviour as an 'illness' and the definition of illness as an undesirable state the issue becomes not *whether* to deal with a particular problem but *how* and *when*. Thus, the debate over homosexuality, drugs, abortion, becomes focussed on the degree of sickness attached to the phenomenon in question or the extent of health risk involved. And the more principled, more perplexing, or even moral issue of *what* freedom should an individual have over his/her own body is shunted aside.

This paper is no attack on medicine as much as on a situation in which we find ourselves in the latter part of the twentieth century. For the medical area is the arena or the example *par excellence* of today's identity crisis – what is or will become of man. It is the battleground not because there are visible threats and oppressors but because they are almost invisible; not because the perspective, tools, and practitioners of medicine and the other helping professions are evil but because they are not. It is so frightening because there are elements here of the banality of evil so uncomfortably written about by Hannah Arendt. But here the danger is greater for not only is the process masked as a technical, scientific, objective one but one done for our own good.

PART X
Doctors and society

measurable terms. The instalments accrue under forms of suffering which exceed the notion of 'pain'.

At some point in the expansion of our major institutions their clients begin to pay a higher price every day for their continued consumption, in spite of the evidence that they will inevitably suffer more. At this point in development the prevalent behaviour of society corresponds to that traditionally recognized in addicts. Declining returns pale in comparison with marginally increasing disutilities. *Homo economicus* turns into *Homo religiosus*. His expectations become heroic. The vengeance of economic development not only outweighs the price at which this vengeance was purchased; it also outweighs the compound tort done by nature and neighbours. Classical nemesis was punishment for the rash abuse of a privilege. Industrialized nemesis is retribution for dutiful participation in society.

War and hunger, pestilence and sudden death, torture and madness remain man's companions, but they are now shaped into a new *Gestalt* by the nemesis overarching them. The greater the economic progress of any community, the greater the part played by industrial nemesis in the pain, discrimination, and death suffered by its members. Therefore, it seems that the disciplined study of the distinctive character of nemesis ought to be the key theme for research among those who are concerned with health care, healing, and consoling.

Tantalus

Medical nemesis is but one aspect of the more general 'counter-intuitive misadventures' characteristic of industrial society. It is the monstrous outcome of a very specific dream of reason-namely, 'tantalising' hubris. Tantalus was a famous king whom the gods invited to Olympus to share one of their meals. He purloined ambrosia, the divine potion which gave the gods unending life. For punishment, he was made immortal in Hades and condemned to suffer unending thirst and hunger. When he bows towards the river in which he stands, the water recedes, and when he reaches for the fruit above his head the branches move out of his reach. Ethologists might say that hygienic nemesis has programmed him for compulsory counter-intuitive be-haviour. Craving for ambrosia has now spread to the common mortal. Scientific and political optimism have combined to propagate the addiction. To sustain it, the priesthood of Tantalus has organized itself, offering unlimited medical improvement of human health. The members of this guild pass themselves off as disciples of healing Aesculapius, while in fact they peddle ambrosia. People demand of them that life be improved, prolonged, rendered compatible with machines, and capable of surviving all modes of acceleration, distortion, and stress. As a result, health has become scarce to the degree to which the common man makes health depend upon the consumption of ambrosia.

Culture and health

Mankind evolved only because each of its individuals came into existence protected by various visible and invisible cocoons. Each one knew the womb from which he had come, and oriented himself by the stars under which he was born. To be human and to become human, the individual of our species has to find his destiny in his unique struggle with nature and neighbour. He is on his own in the struggle, but the weapons and the rules and the style are given to him by the culture in which he grew up. Each culture is the sum of rules with which the individual could come to terms with pain, sickness, and death – could interpret them and practise compassion among others faced by the same threats. Each culture set the myth, the rituals, the taboos, and the ethical standards needed to deal with the fragility of life – to explain the reason for pain, the dignity of the sick, and the role of dying or death.

Cosmopolitan medical civilization denies the need for man's acceptance of these evils. Medical civilization is planned and organized to kill pain, to eliminate sickness, and to struggle against death. These are new goals, which have never before been guidelines for social life and which are antithetic to every one of the cultures with which medical civilization meets when it is dumped on the so-called poor as part and parcel of their economic progress.

The health-denying effect of medical civilization is thus equally powerful in rich and in poor countries, even though the latter are often spared some of its more sinister sides.

The killing of pain

For an experience to be pain in the full sense, it must fit into a culture. Precisely because each culture provides a mode for suffering, culture is a particular form of health. The act of suffering is shaped by culture into a question which can be stated and shared.

Medical civilization replaces the culturally determined competence in suffering with a growing demand by each individual for the institutional management of his pain. A myriad of different feelings, each expressing some kind of fortitude, are homogenized into the political pressure of anaesthesia consumers. Pain becomes an item on a list of complaints. As a result, a new kind of horror emerges. Conceptually it is still pain, but the impact on our emotions of this valueless, opaque, and impersonal hurt is something quite new.

In this way, pain has come to pose only a technical question for industrial man – what do I need to get in order to have my pain managed or killed? By becoming unnecessary, pain has become unbearable. With this attitude, it now seems rational to flee pain rather than to face it, even at the cost of addiction. It also seems reasonable to eliminate pain, even at the cost of health. It seems enlightened to deny legitimacy to all non-technical issues which pain raises, even at the cost of disarming the victims of residual pain. For a while it can be argued that the total pain anaesthetized in a society is greater than the totality of pain newly generated. But at some point, rising marginal disutilities set in. The new suffering is not only unmanageable, but it has lost its referential character. It has become meaningless, questionless torture. Only the recovery of the will and ability to suffer can restore health into pain.

The elimination of sickness

Medical interventions have not affected total mortality rates; at best they have shifted survival from one segment of the population to another. Dramatic changes in the nature of disease afflicting Western societies during the last hundred years are well documented. First industrialization exacerbated infections, which then subsided. Tuberculosis peaked over a fifty to seventy-five-year period and declined before either the tubercle bacillus had been discovered or anti-tuberculous programmes had been initiated. It was replaced in Britain and the USA by major malnutrition syndromes – rickets and pellagra – which peaked and declined, to be replaced by disease of early childhood, which in turn gave way to duodenal ulcers in young men. When that declined the modern epidemics took their toll – coronary heart-disease, hypertension, cancer, arthritis, diabetes, and mental disorders. At least in the USA, death rates from hypertensive heart-disease seem to be declining. Despite intensive research no connection between these changes in disease patterns can be attributed to the professional practice of medicine.

Neither decline in any of the major epidemics of killing diseases, nor major changes in the age structure of the population, nor falling and rising absenteeism at the workbench have been significantly related to sick care – even to immunization. Medical services deserve neither credit for longevity nor blame for the threatening population pressure.

Longevity owes much more to the railroad and to the synthesis of fertilizers and insecticides than it owes to new drugs and syringes. Professional practice is both ineffective and increasingly sought out. This technically unwarranted rise of medical prestige can only be explained as a magical ritual for the achievement of goals which are beyond technical and political reach. It can be countered only through legislation and political action which favours the deprofessionalization of health care.

The overwhelming majority of modern diagnostic and therapeutic interventions which demonstrably do more good than harm have two characteristics: the material resources for them are extremely cheap, and they can be packaged and designed for self-use or application by family members. The price of technology that is significantly health furthering or curative in Canadian medicine is so low that the resources now squandered in India on modern medicine would suffice to make it available in the entire sub-continent. On the other hand, the skills needed for the application of the most generally used diagnostic and therapeutic aids are so simple that the careful observation of instruction by people who personally care would guarantee more effective and responsible use than medical practice can provide.

The deprofessionalization of medicine does not imply and should not be read as implying negation of specialized healers, of competence, of mutual criticism, or of public control. It does imply a bias against mystification, against transnational dominance of one orthodox view, against disbarment of healers chosen by their patients but not certified by the guild. The deprofessionalization of medicine does not mean denial of public funds for curative purposes; it does mean a bias against the disbursement of any such funds under the prescription and control of guild members, rather than under the control of the consumer. Deprofessionalization does not mean the elimination of modern medicine, nor obstacles to the invention of new ones, nor necessarily the return to ancient programmes, rituals, and devices. It means that no professional shall have the power to lavish on any one of his patients a package of curative resources larger than that which any other could claim on his own. Finally, the deprofessionalization of medicine does not mean disregard for the special needs which people manifest at special moments of their lives; when they are born, break a leg, marry, give birth, become crippled, or face death. It only means that people have a right to live in an environment which is hospitable to them at such high points of experience.

The struggle against death

The ultimate effect of medical nemesis is the expropriation of death. In every society the image of death is the culturally conditioned anticipation of an uncertain date. This anticipation determines a series of behavioural norms during life and the structure of certain institutions.

Wherever modern medical civilization has penetrated a traditional medical culture, a novel cultural ideal of death has been fostered. The new ideal spreads by means of technology and the professional ethos which corresponds to it.

We cannot fully understand contemporary social organization unless we see in it a multi-faceted exorcism of all forms of evil death. Our major institutions constitute a gigantic defence programme waged on behalf of 'humanity' against all those people who can be associated with what is currently conceived of as death-dealing social injustice. Not only medical agencies, but welfare, international relief, and development programmes are enlisted in this struggle. Ideological bureaucracies of all colours join the crusade. Even war has been used to justify the defeat of those who are blamed for wanton tolerance of sickness and death. Producing 'natural death' for all is at the point of becoming an ultimate justification for social control. Under the influence of medical rituals contemporary death is again the rationale for a witch-hunt.

Conclusion

Rising irreparable damage accompanies industrial expansion in all sectors. In medicine these damages appear as iatrogenesis. Iatrogenesis can be direct, when pain, sickness, and death result from medical care, or it can be indirect, when health policies reinforce an industrial organization which generates ill health; it can be structural when medically sponsored behaviour and delusion restrict the vital autonomy of people by undermining their competence in growing up, caring, ageing, or when it nullifies the personal challenge arising from their pain, disability, and anguish.

Most of the remedies proposed to reduce iatrogenesis are engineering interventions. They are therapeutically designed in their approach to the individual, the group, the institution, or the environment. These so-called remedies generate second-order iatrogenic ills by creating a new prejudice against the autonomy of the citizen.

The most profound iatrogenic effects of the medical technostructure result from its non-technical social functions. The sickening technical and non-technical consequences of the institutionalization of medicine coalesce to generate a new kind of suffering – anaesthetized and solitary survival in a world-wide hospital ward.

Medical nemesis cannot be operationally verified. Much less can it be measured. The intensity with which it is experienced depends on the independence, vitality, and relatedness of each individual. As a theoretical concept it is one component in a broad theory to explain the anomalies plaguing health-care systems in our day. It is an aspect of an even more general phenomenon which I have called industrial nemesis, the backlash of institutionally structured industrial hubris. This hubris consists of a disregard for the boundaries within which the human phenomenon remains visible. Current research is overwhelmingly oriented towards unattainable 'breakthroughs'. What I have called counterfoil research is the disciplined analysis of the levels at which such reverberations must inevitably damage man.

The perception of enveloping nemesis leads to a social choice. Either the natural boundaries of human endeavour are estimated, recognized, and translated into politically determined limits, or the alternative to extinction is compulsory survival in a planned and engineered hell.

Man's consciously lived fragility, individuality, and relatedness make the experience of pain, of sickness, and of death an integral part of his life. The ability to cope with this trio in autonomy is fundamental to his health. To the degree to which he becomes dependent on the management of his intimacy he renounces his autonomy and his health *must* decline. The true miracle of modern medicine is diabolical. It consists of making not only individuals but whole populations survive on inhumanly low levels of personal health. That health should decline with increasing health-service delivery is unforeseen only by the health manager, precisely because his strategies are the result of his blindness to the inalienability of health.

The level of public health corresponds to the degree to which the means and responsibility for coping with illness are distributed among the total population. This ability to cope can be enhanced but never replaced by medical intervention in the lives of people or the hygienic characteristics of the environment. That society which can reduce professional intervention to the minimum will provide the best conditions for health. The greater the potential for autonomous adaptation to self and to others and to the environment, the less management of adaptation will be needed or tolerated.

The recovery of a healthy attitude towards sickness is neither Luddite nor romantic nor Utopian: it is a guiding ideal which will never be fully achieved, but which must orient politics to avoid encroaching nemesis.

30 Health – a demystification of medical technology

Halfdan Mahler*

[*This paper has been edited from the original in accordance with the editors' general strategy. The author is Director-General of the World Health Organization.*]

The mystery holders

The wave of social consciousness in the nineteenth century in Europe and in North America broadened our understanding of 'Health' but resulted in a reaction by the medical establishment and a constriction which is still continuing. By legislation, by training, by organization, and by the way in which health-related interventions are stated and restricted, there has been a progressive 'mystification' in medical care which is continuing almost unchecked. As our understanding of cause and effect has grown, 'medicine' has continued to restrict the range of problems for which it considers itself responsible and the gap between 'health care' and 'medical care' has become ever wider. This has been coupled with an organizational change which has influenced the manner

* extracted from an inaugural lecture of the British Postgraduate Medical Federation's 1975–76 Scientific Basis of Medicine series, delivered in London on Oct. 9. Reprinted in the *Lancet* (1975): 829–33, November 1.

of dealing with these problems, a gross restriction in the information available and decisions to be made by people outside the health professions, and an unnecessary but inevitable dependency of the population upon the holders of these mysteries.

If true, this is a grave charge. As with all such general charges the evidence adds up to suspicion rather than certainty. If one looks back to the last century in England, the attack upon some of the physical evils of the Industrial Revolution was clearly led by social reformers, such as the Chadwicks, the health professions having secondary roles such as certifying most questionably the health effects of rising damp and back-to-back houses. There was a change in the disease picture (especially the communicable diseases) but the evidence linking this to medical improvement interventions rather than to changes in the society and the environment is also questionable. The continuing decreases in incidence and mortality appear to be largely extensions of continuing trends and were not directly related, in time, to immunization or to direct medical action.

Parallel to these changes in disease pictures came a change in distribution of health resources. On the one hand there was the expansion of coverage to the universality of access which one now has, and on the other came the increased expenditure of specialized resources upon the few. This meant that a widening of the base did not result in a lowering of the peak or a flattening of the health expenditure pyramid. The peak is still rising higher, but this time it is a peak of expenditure directed towards the few, selected not so much by social class or wealth but by medical technology itself. Such an evolution is a world-wide rather than a peculiarly national trend. In some places where it has been examined it has been identified as an increasing expenditure upon persons in the final months or years before death. It appears that this expenditure does not measurably increase life expectancy or make humanly tolerable the closing episodes of the lives of elderly people. In other countries the increased expenditure on the few has been linked to the 'upgrading' of health care interventions to higher and higher levels of the medical establishment. This is typified by a statement of intent, within a developing country with a high maternal and neonatal mortality, that the medium-term objective will be to arrange that every woman in labour should be delivered by a consultant specialist obstetrician. Many other examples of the same trend can be cited. When added together they appear to say that health workers consider that the 'best' health care is one where everything known to medicine is applied to every individual, by the most highly trained medical scientist, in the most specialized institution. This type of thinking is clearly as dangerous as it would be for me, who spends so much time flying from Member State to Member State, if I preferred the aircraft in which I was travelling to be flown by a professor of aeronautical engineering rather than by an experienced pilot.

If one follows this same line of thought one understands the inevitable side effect that, as health care action moves higher and higher up the referral ladder, it comes to be justified more and more by the actions themselves and is more restricted. It is frightening but expected that when a specialized group is formed to perform certain actions it is evaluated and continues to be supported because of the *number* of such actions which it does, rather than by whether a problem is solved. There are counter-reactions to such trends well typified by the recent public debate over the treatment of spina bifida. Another example of reaction to this path could be a children's burn unit in a major city which showed that many of its intake of cases resulted from injuries caused by scalding coffee in the home. Rather than conducting research upon a more effective treatment of burns it directed its attention to the design of a coffee-pot which would not spill. The wide acceptance of the new design led to a decreased number of cases. But these exceptions make existing trends even more frightening.

Such trends towards restricted high technology might be said to be a by-product of medical research distortions, and a good case might be made for directing a portion of the blame to the priorities of research workers supported for the most part from national funds. But such finger pointing cannot explain all that is happening. The movements of interventions further up the professional ladder and the increased restriction of action to fewer and fewer people do not seem to be related only to new research findings. The implications of such a movement are not only seen as an increase in costs with few measurable health advantages in terms of either morbidity and mortality: they are also seen as a downgrading in social status of health workers at the bottom of the pyramid, changing aspirations of health workers who understand-ably want to be legitimized to as high a point in the pyramid as possible, or public reaction such as the disturbances in the United States of America caused by the increase in malpractice litigation.

Four questions

What I have been describing is not a single, simple, phenomenon of our time but a complex of events. Some of the elements of this complex might become clearer if phrased as four questions:

(1) Is it possible to assign health resources within a country on a problem-solving basis (using different mixes of preventive curative, promotive, and rehabilitative action)?

(2) What medical interventions are truly effective and specific for prevention, treatment, or rehabilitation, as measured in objective terms?

(3) Can such medical interventions and the risk groups to which they should be applied be described objectively and in such a manner that the amount of skill and knowledge required for their application can be assessed?

(4) Is it possible to design a health care establishment to carry out the above tasks which will result in the most meaningful interventions reaching the greatest proportion of persons at risk, as early as possible, at the least cost, and in an acceptable manner?

There is little doubt that it would be considered reasonable to ask questions of this type if we were dealing with a non-health topic such as education or transportation, and to answer them with a positive reply. In health, persons within the establishment might disagree that the questions are the dominant or relevant ones, or even try to make the case that health is in some way different. Non-health individuals might react differently and even express astonishment at these questions because many may fondly assume that their health services *are* designed to deal with problems; the interventions they pay for *are* known to be effective and appropriate; and the person who is responsible for the medical care they receive *is* the appropriate person in training and position for their needs. Such is not the case.

I am convinced that all of the questions can be answered positively. But this does not mean that, if a country and a health care establishment did assign resources on a problem-solving basis, using methods known to be effective by the most appropriate people to apply them, this would be the perfect health service requiring no further change. Problems change; societies and priorities change, and will keep on changing. Society's instruments for action must keep changing too. New interventions will continue to be evolved as our knowledge and understanding grow. New types of action must lead to changes in the role of health workers. But if change would be needed in the future within a service based upon such principles, it is equally likely that change is needed *now* when we do not have such perfection.

However, countries have pasts as well as futures and the incredible investment of the past in institutions, industries, people, knowledge, and public awareness and acceptance cannot be discarded with a playful laugh. It would be a foolhardy decision-maker who took lightly the risk of discarding what we now have in the hope that what would come next would be better.

But there is some middle ground between those either frightened of any change or confidently proud of present achievements, and the grim and embarrassing rationalists wanting to make a new start because they consider that the present system is an adapted historical accident, unjustifiable on any grounds, and following its own professional path divorced from people's needs.

Objective measurement

The entry point in my view are my questions two and three. Techniques already exist to examine medical technology and to express in objective terms what works, whether it matters, and what it costs. The studies on such subjects have been of three types.

The first are cold, planned, controlled clinical trials testing whether intervention A gives a better result than intervention B. Such clinical trials are medical extensions of the scientific method; their mechanics are widely known, and both their conduct and their results give satisfactions to both the investigators and the consumers.

The second type of study is much more rare and is not greeted with such universal approval. A good example is the study of anaemia in the United Kingdom where the questions were: What is anaemia? What level of haemoglobin really matters? and how effective is the treatment to persons below this level? So much of ill health as we now see it is not divided from the normal by a clear division point; yet establishing where the dividing line rests not only is of concern to millions of individuals, but also, if it can be related to outcomes, can save huge amounts of money and man-hours of work, and false explanations to patients with complaints...

There are even fewer examples of the third type of study. These are trials which require the results of the previous two trials as their starting point. They start from a dialogue between the national medical establishment and the national government which recommends that at this time, and from evidence provided by trials such as the above, such-and-such a health problem is relevant and important and this-or-that intervention to a certain part of the population could be the best national strategy. From this decision trials could be designed to see how this could best be done on the grounds of cost, efficiency, and acceptability ... Some such trials are multi-staged; the provincial trials in

Mexico aimed at decreasing deaths in infants from diarrhoeal disease are a case in point. Here a review of the evidence clearly pointed to dehydration as the immediate main cause of death, and the first trials based upon district rehydration centres were clearly effective in decreasing mortality. But rehydration centres were also expensive, required specialized staff, needed transport systems to the inaccessible villages, and had the image of high technology brought to bear on what is understood as a household problem. The next phase of the trials was the preparation and testing of salts for rehydration in such a form that they could be produced cheaply, prepared and used by anyone including the mother, and distributed through existing networks. This proved to be equally effective, much cheaper, and highly acceptable ... Many trials of this type have been directed at rare rather than common problems, and some of the results have been rejected or the findings have not been applied. I suspect that this has sometimes been because the medical establishment plus its efficient medical lobby have considered that the necessary health service changes would either decrease or change their influence, their status, or their incomes. The public outcry, when the subject has been one of public debate, has been on the grounds that there will be a decrease in the 'quality' of service. 'Quality' is a dangerous argument to make in a health service which is not problem oriented but institution oriented. As the public becomes increasingly aware that different drugs – all of which have been monitored for national standards of safety and efficacy and which are similar in all relevant respects except price – are being prescribed for the same condition, it is highly likely that such examples of apparent rejection of a successful trial will be used against the medical establishment as a whole.

I strongly advocate a massive encouragement of all three types of trials and I consider that, while these have been largely completed in my particular field of tuberculosis, there are enormous gaps in many other problem areas. As the World Health Organization responds to requests from governments for assistance at the periphery, we are aware that at the village level a considerable proportion of the interventions have not been examined in this way. We suspect that at the district hospital and health centre level the proportion is at least as great.

Claim for diversity

While there may be little disagreement that medical interventions or technology need to be tested objectively and that this testing should continue to the population-based problem level, I am aware of implications which require further discussion. It is reasonable to ask whether, if such testing is completed with the best of our presently available knowledge and gives a meaningful result, this answer should be a national or a world standard and whether all of us should conform to it. If a country makes a different decision, will it be providing or advocating a lower 'quality' of care? The answer to both these questions must be no for two different reasons. First, both the importance and the nature of problems vary from place to place, and from country to country. A good example of this is the different responses to oral poliomyelitis vaccine in tropical and temperate zones. But, even after putting these important arguments to one side, there are good reasons for advocating national rather than international decisions. If I return to the diarrhoeal disease example I mentioned earlier, the result of providing rehydration centres, of distributing simple home-based rehydration fluids, or of possibly improving the environment and decreasing faecal-oral transmission or assisting families to provide their children with an adequate diet, may all be the same. All may result in a clear decrease in deaths from diarrhoeal disease. Some may have other positive or negative effects as well such as decreasing diarrhoeal incidence or decreasing the likelihood of dying from measles. Each may have a different cost. All of these variations are important and need to be taken into account when a decision is made; but it cannot be said that a country which decides upon rehydration by the mother has taken a decision to give a lower quality of service than the one which will build rehydration centres staffed by doctors or nurses. I can think of major disadvantages of discouraging diversity between countries in the same way that there must be omissions, waste, and dangers through not having a national decision-making process within countries or regions to answer and decide upon such questions.

The collection of evidence which can be used to decide what is our problem-based health technology opens great opportunities of research for the individual research worker, for professional groups, and for governments. This is research in the broadest sense and need be no poor and low-class relation to other research aimed at increasing fundamental knowledge of our biomedical world. And this type of research would make major contributions to the demystification of medical technology.

Starting points for change

Up to this point I consider that what I have said should not be in major conflict with the main lines of world medical thought – although in deep conflict with actual delivery of health care. However, I wish to make two further points which are more speculative and are much more an expression of my views upon the world and society than upon medical technology.

The first is that, while health services are clearly an integral part of a country's social policy and political structure, we must assume that health policies and actions can be changed and improved without a change in the basis of government. If this is possible, and if a government considers that health is a basic right of each member of its population, then a change to a more efficient, acceptable, and just health system can be made by concentrating upon and answering the three final questions I have already given. I am conscious of the number of 'ifs' I must make in this statement and the few examples I can show to base it upon. Much of my conviction must come by analogy from other sectors where the starting point for progressive change has been an agreement upon the nature and the extent of the problem followed by an objective assessment of what can be done about it, thus avoiding subjugating the problem to technology. I consider that agreement upon the usefulness, practicability, and ranking of this priority step would be a major advance. We all know that there are serious defects in the health systems of many countries and we must have a starting point for change. One such point suggested frequently is a change in the education and training of health workers, but there have been no clear successes using this strategy. It has proved easier for health workers to adapt to the existing system, even when they are trained for different tasks, than to change the system itself. Another purposed starting point has been centralized planning. While this has resulted in documented successes, these have frequently been where the problems have been clear (such as epidemic disease) and the interventions equally clear. What I am advocating, for the industrial as well as the developing world, is for the health establishment to make a major effort to describe all the health problems and the alternative ways of dealing with them in an objective way and then to accept a national decision process based upon this evidence. Such a series of steps has risks as well as advantages and assumes both a level of scientific detachment which is clearly obvious to all and an acceptance that the final decisions are made by society rather than by the concerned professionals.

My final point has two parts and is equally speculative. The first is that it makes good social, economic, and professional sense for countries to take the choice of intervention options nearer to the consumer whenever they have the chance. If I use my diarrhoeal disease example, I would say that making rehydration salts for babies available to mothers in every home is likely to be more useful in the short, medium, and long term than expecting the mother to take the baby to a special centre and have this service done for her. There should be no secret either in the way in which diarrhoeal disease occurs or in its treatment. There appears to be no possible reason why the knowledge and the skills of dealing with it should not go down the professional tree to every household at risk. This is what I mean by 'demystification' of medical technology.

There are other possibilities of reversing the trend which is pushing medical action higher up the professional tree. Surely there are immediate opportunities of shifting action downwards at least one step – from teaching hospitals to regional hospitals, from consultants to general practitioners, from general practitioners to nurses, from nurses to mothers? Such a process has to be undertaken carefully and with real understanding. I am well aware of the apparent relationship between, for example, those areas in Europe which have moved from domiciliary to institutional deliveries and a decreasing maternal and neonatal mortality. Which factors have influenced these changes have never been clarified but the relationship may well be real. The indicators of success in a reverse move aimed at other problems may be very different ones from deaths. Possibly we could expect similar figures for disease and death but rising indices expressing satisfaction and understanding, a decrease in costs, and a larger population group who will have this service. And it is this larger population participation that eventually might open the doors to effective prevention of, for example, cancer and cardiovascular diseases. Indeed it could bring us closer to WHO's constitutional objective: the attainment by all peoples of the highest possible level of physical, mental, and social well-being and not merely the absence of disease or infirmity.

If such indices matter as objectives as well as methods of measurement, there are other implications. They must also influence the studies upon the definition of health technology which I mentioned earlier. They may be one more factor, even the dominant factor, in deciding what is important or relevant as well as who should have the responsibility for action.

Conclusion

The medical establishment is in real trouble. Not only is it caught in the worries of rising costs versus finite budgets but it has the problem of defining its own image and philosophy. In our present world, 'high technology' is no longer thought of as the description of 'what is possible' – whether this be in atomic power or voyages to the moon. Now it must be the assistance in reaching certain goals under quite clearly defined conditions. We must simply state what we can do, so that all can understand, and then help to design a service based upon society's values, and with a human face. I am confident that it can be done, if we want to do it – and the United Kingdom has indeed demonstrated a good deal of pragmatic vigour in this respect. But I am sceptical that we are anything near the critical mass of professional desire to stop confusing health with conventional medical wisdom. If this scepticism proves correct, then we can look forward to a long period of confrontation before anything like the dialogue I have proposed can begin.

References

References

ALINSKY, S. (1967) The Poor and the Powerful. In *Poverty and Mental Health*. Psychiatric Research Reports No. 21 of the American Psychiatric Association, January.

ANDERSON, J., DAY, D. L., DOWLING, M. A. C., and PETTINGALE, K. W. (1970) The Definition and Evaluation of the Skills Required to Obtain a Patient's History of Illness: The Use of Videotape Recordings. *Post-Graduate Medical Journal* 46: 606.

ASHFORD, J. R. and PEARSON, N.G. (1970) Who Uses the Health Services and Why? *Journal of the Royal Statistical Society Series A: General 133*, part 3: 295.

ATCHLEY, R. C. (1970) A Qualification of Test Factor Standardization: A Methodological Note. *Social Forces* 49: 84–5.

BAKWIN, H. (1945) Pseudocia pediatricia. New England Journal of Medicine 232: 691–7.

BALINT, ENID and NORRELL, J. S. (1973) *Six Minutes for the Patient*. London: Tavistock Publications.

BALINT, MICHAEL (1957) *The Doctor, his Patient, and the Illness*. London: Pitman Medical. See Reading 15.

————— and BALINT, ENID (1961) *Psychotherapeutic Techniques in Medicine*. London: Tavistock Publications.

—————, —————, GOSLING, R., and HILDEBRAND, P. (1966) *A Study of Doctors*. London: Tavistock Publications.

—————, JOYCE, D., MARINKER, M., and WOODCOCK, J. (1970) *Treatment or Diagnosis: A Study of Repeat Prescribing in General Practice*. London: Tavistock Publications.

BANKS, MICHAEL H., BERESFORD, S. A. A., MORRELL, D. C., WALLER, J. J., and WATKINS, C. J. (1975) Factors Influencing the Demand for Primary Medical Care in Women aged 20–44 Years: A Preliminary Report. *International Journal of Epidemiology* 4(3): 189–95. See Reading 13.

BECK, A. T. (1967) *Depression: Clinical, Experimental and Theoretical Aspects*. New York: Harper & Row.

BECKER, E. (1962) Towards a Comprehensive Theory of Depression. *Journal of Nervous and Mental Diseases* 135: 26–35.

BLACKWELL, B. (1963) The Literature of Delay in Seeking Medical Care for Chronic Illness. *Health Education Monographs* 16: 3–32.

BLALOCK, H. M. (1960) *Social Statistics*. New York: McGraw-Hill.

————— (1964) Controlling for Background Factors: Spuriousness versus Developmental Sequences. *Social Enquiry* 34: 28–40.

BOZEMAN, M. F., ORBACH, C. E., and SUTHERLAND, A. M. (1955) Psychological Impact of Cancer and its Treatment, III. The Adaptation of Mothers to the Threatened Loss of their Children through Leukemia. Part I. *Cancer* 8: 1.

BRILL, N. Q. and STORROW, H. A. (1964) Social Class and Psychiatric Treatment. In F. Riessman, J. Cohen, and A. Pearl (eds.), *Mental Health of the Poor*. New York: The Free Press.

BRITISH MEDICAL JOURNAL (1976) 1 1362.

BROWN, GEORGE W. (1973) Some Thoughts on Grounded Theory. *Sociology* 7(1): 1–16.

————— (1976) Depression: A Sociological View. *The Maudsley Gazette*: 9–12, Summer. See Reading 25.

—————, BIRLEY, J. L. T., and WING, JOHN K. (1972) Influence of Family Life on the Course of Schizophrenic Disorders: A Replication. *British Journal of Psychiatry* 121: 241–58. See Reading 8.

—————, HARRIS, TIRRIL, and NÍ BHROLCHÁIN, MAIRE (1975) Social Class and Psychiatric Disturbance among Women in an Urban Population. *Sociology* 9: 225–54.

—————, HARRIS, TIRRIL, and PETO, J. (1973) Life Events and Psychiatric Disorder: 2 Nature of Causal Link. *Psychological Medicine* 3(2): 159–76.

—————, MONCK, E. M., CARSTAIRS, G. M., and WING, JOHN K. (1962) The Influence of Family Life on the Course of Schizophrenic Illness. *British Journal of Preventive and Social Medicine* 16: 55.

————— and RUTTER, MICHAEL, L. (1966) The Measurement of Family Activities and Relationships. *Human Relations* 19: 241–63. See Reading 1.

BUCHAN, I. C. and RICHARDSON, I. M. (1973) *Time Study of Consultations in General Practice*. Scottish Health Studies No. 27, Scottish Home and Health Department.

BUXTON, M. J. and KLEIN, R. E. (1975) Division of Hospital Provision: Policy Themes and Resource Variations. *British Medical Journal Supplement* i: 354–59.

CAMERON, A. and HINTON, J. (1968) Delay in Seeking Treatment for Mammary Tumours. *Cancer* 21: 1121–126.

CARTWRIGHT, ANN (1964) *Human Relations and Hospital Care.* London: Routledge & Kegan Paul.

———— (1967) *Patients and their doctors.* London: Routledge & Kegan Paul.

———— (1970) *Parents and Family Planning Services.* London: Routledge & Kegan Paul.

————, LUCAS, SUSAN, and O'BRIEN, MAUREEN (1974) Exploring Communication in General Practice. Report to the Social Science Research Council.

———— and O'BRIEN, MAUREEN (1976) Social Class Variations in Health Care and in the Nature of General Practice Consultations. In M. Stacey (ed.), *The Sociology of the National Health Service. Sociological Review* Monograph No. 22. Keele: University of Keele. See Reading 10.

CASSEL, J. (1967) Factors Involving Sociocultural Incongruity and Change: Appraisal and Implications for Theoretical Development. *Millbank Memorial Fund Quarterly* XLV(2) part 2: 41–8, April.

CHAPMAN, W. P. and JONES, C. H. (1944) Variations in Cutaneous and Visceral Pain Sensitivity in Normal Subjects. *Journal of Clinical Investigation* 23: 81.

COMMISSION ON CHRONIC ILLNESS (1957) *Chronic Illness in a Large City.* Cambridge, Mass.: Harvard University Press.

COOPER, J. E. (1970) The Use of a Procedure for Standardizing Psychiatric Diagnosis. In E. H. Hare and John K. Wing (eds.), *Psychiatric Epidemiology.* London: Oxford University Press.

COSER, ROSE LAUB (1964) Alienation and the Social Structure. In Eliot Freidson (ed.), *The Hospital in Modern Society.* New York: The Free Press. See Reading 24.

DAVIS, FRED (1956) Definitions of Time and Recovery in Paralytic Polio Convalescence. *American Journal of Sociology* LXI: 582–87, May.

———— (1960) Uncertainty in Medical Prognosis: Clinical and Functional. *American Journal of Sociology* 66: 41–7. See Reading 17.

DE LEVITA, D. J. (1958) From *Tijdschrift voor Sociale Geneeskunde* 36: 200.

DINGWALL, ROBERT, HEATH, CHRISTIAN, REID, MARGARET, and STACEY, MARGARET (eds.) (1977) *Health Care and Health Knowledge.* London: Croom Helm.

DUBOS, R. (1959) *The Mirage of Health.* Garden City, New York: Doubleday.

———— (1965) *Man Adapting.* New Haven: Yale University Press.

DUNNELL, KAREN and CARTWRIGHT, ANN (1972) *Medicine Takers, Prescribers and Horders.* London: Routledge & Kegan Paul.

DURKHEIM, E. (Trans. 1952) *Suicide.* London: Routledge & Kegan Paul.

EGBERT, LAWRENCE D., BATTIT, GEORGE E., WELCH, CLAUDE E., and BARTLETT, MICHAEL K. (1964) Reduction of Postoperative Pain by Encouragement and Instruction of Patients. *The New England Journal of Medicine* 270: 825–27. See Reading 20.

EISENBERG, L. (1966) Genetics and the Survival of the Unfit. *Harper's Magazine* **232**: 57.

ENGEL, G. L. (1961) Is Grief a Disease? A Challenge for Medical Research. *Psychosomatic Medicine* **23**(18): 4.

EPSOM, JOSEPH E. (1969) The Mobile Health Clinic: A Report on the First Year's Work. Mimeo from the London Borough of Southwark Health Department. See Reading 12.

FENICHEL, O. (1946) *The Psycho-Analytic Theory of the Neuroses*. London: Routledge & Kegan Paul.

FISHER, RONALD A. (1947) *The Design of Experiments*. Edinburgh: Oliver & Boyd.

FLEISS, J. L. (1973) *Statistical Methods for Rates and Proportions*. New York: John Wiley & Sons, Inc.

FOX, RENEE (1957) Training for Uncertainty. In R. K. Merton, G. Reader, and P. L. Kendall (eds.), *The Student-Physician*. Cambridge, Mass.: Harvard University Press.

FREIDSON, ELIOT (1960) Client Control and Medical Practice. *American Journal of Sociology* **65**: 374–82.

——— (1964) *The Hospital in Modern Society*. New York: The Free Press.

——— (1970) *Professions of Medicine*. New York: Dodd, Mead & Co.

FRIEDMAN, STANFORD BARTON, CHODOFF, PAUL, MASON, JOHN W., and HAMBURG, DAVID A. (1963) Behavioral Observations on Parents Anticipating the Death of a Sick Child. *Pediatrics* **32**: 610–25. See Reading 9.

GARLAND, L. H. (1959) Studies on the Accuracy of Diagnostic Procedures. *American Journal of Roentgenology, Radium Therapy, and Nuclear Medicine* **82**: 25–38.

GEERTSEN, H. R. and GRAY, R. M. (1970) Familistic Orientation and Inclination towards Adopting the Sick Role. *Journal of Marriage and the Family* **32**: 638.

GLASER, BARNEY G. and STRAUSS, ANSELM L. (1968) *The Discovery of Grounded Theory: Strategies for Qualitative Research*. London: Weidenfeld and Nicolson.

GOFFMAN, ERVING (1968) *Asylums*. Harmondsworth: Penguin.

GOLDBERG, D. P. and BLACKWELL, B. (1970) Psychiatric Illness in General Practice – A Detailed Study Using a New Method of Case Identification. *British Medical Journal* ii: 439.

GOLDHAMER, H. and MARSHALL, A. W. (1949) *Psychosis and Civilization*. Glencoe, Illinois: The Free Press.

GREEN, W. A. JR and MILLER, G. (1958) Psychological Factors and Reticuloendothelial Disease IV. Observations on a Group of Children and Adolescents with Leukemia: An Interpretation of Disease Development in terms of the Mother–Child Unit. *Psychosomatic Medicine* **20**: 124.

HAMPTON, J. R., HARRIS, M. J. G, MITCHELL, J. R. A., PRITCHARD, J. S., and SEYMOUR, C. (1975) The Relative Contributions of History-taking, Physical Examination and Laboratory Investigations to the Diagnosis and Management of Medical Outpatients. *British Medical Journal* ii: 486.

HANNAY, D. R. (1972) Accuracy of Health Centre Records. *Lancet* ii: 371.

HARDY, J. D., WOLFF, H. G., and GOODELL, H. (1952) *Pain Sensations and Reactions*. Baltimore: Williams and Wilkins.

HART, JULIAN TUDOR (1971) The Inverse Care Law. *Lancet* i: 405–12.

——— (1972) Data on Occupational Mortality 1959–63. *Lancet* i: 192–93.

HILL, A. BRADFORD (1950) *Principles of Medical Statistics*. London: Lancet.

——— (ed.) (1960) *Controlled Clinical Trials*. Springfield, Illinois: Charles C. Thomas.

HMSO (1974) Office of Population Censuses and Surveys: Morbidity Statistics from General Practice, Studies on Medical and Population Subjects No. 26.

HOFFMAN, M. L. (1960) Power Assertion by the Parent and its Impact on the Child. *Child Development* 31: 129–43.

HOLLINGSHEAD, A. B. and REDLICH, F. C. (1958) *Social Class and Mental Illness: A Community Study*. New York: John Wiley.

HORDER, J. and HORDER, E. (1954) *Illness in General Practice*. The *Practitioner* 173.

HUGHES, E. C. (1958) *Men and their Work*. New York: The Free Press.

HULL, F. M. (1969) Social Class Consultation Patterns in Rural General Practice. *The Journal of the Royal College of General Practitioners* 18: 65.

ILLICH, IVAN (1971a) *Deschooling Society*. London: Marion Boyars.

——— (1971b) *Celebration of Awareness*. London: Marion Boyars.

——— (1973) *Tools for Conviviality*. London: Marion Boyars.

——— (1974a) Medical Nemesis. *Lancet* i: 918–21, May 11. See Reading 29.

——— (1974b) *Energy and Equity*. London: Marion Boyars.

——— (1976) *Limits to Medicine. Medical Nemesis: The Expropriation of Health*. London: Marion Boyars.

——— (1977) *Disabling Professions*. London: Marion Boyars.

JANIS, I. L. (1958) *Psychological Stress: Psychoanalytic and Behavioral Studies of Surgical Patients*. New York: John Wiley & Sons, Inc.

JEFFERYS, MARGOT (1974) Does Medicine Need Sociology? *The University of London Bulletin* No. 6: 7–9, March. See Reading 5.

KASL, S. V. and COBB, S. (1966) Health Behaviour, Illness Behaviour and Sick Role Behaviour. *Archives of Environmental Health* 12: 246.

KEDWARD, H. B. (1962) Social Class Habits of Consulting. *British Journal of Preventive and Social Medicine* 16: 147.

KEYS, A. (1972) The Epidemiology of Coronary Heart Disease. *Cardiovascular Epidemiology Newsletter*: 2–5.

KORSCH, B. M., GOZZI, E. K., and FRANCIS, V. (1968) Gaps in Doctor–Patient Communications. *Pediatrics* 42: 855.

KUTNER, BERNARD (1958) Surgeons and their Patients. In E. Gartly Jaco (ed.), *Patients, Physicians and Illness*. Glencoe, Illinois: The Free Press.

LASAGNA, L. and BEECHER, H. K. (1954) Analgesic Effectiveness of Codeine and Meperidine (Demerol). *Journal of Pharmacology and Experimental Therapeutics* 112: 306–11.

LAZARSFELD, P. and ROSENBERG, MORRIS (eds.) (1955) *The Language of Social Research*. Glencoe, Illinois: The Free Press.

LEFF, JULIAN P. and WING, JOHN K. (1971) Trial of Maintenance Therapy in Schizophrenia. *British Medical Journal* 3: 599–604.

LEIFER, R. (1969) *In the Name of Mental Health*. New York: Science House.

LEMERT, E. M. (1951) *Social Pathology*. New York: McGraw-Hill.

LEONARD, ROBERT C., SKIPPER, JAMES K., and WOOLRIDGE, P. (1967) Small Sample Field Experiments for Evaluating Patient Care. *Health Services Research* 2 (Spring): 46–60.

L'ETANG, H. (1970) *The Pathology of Leadership*. New York: Hawthorne Books.

LIBERMAN, R. P. and RASKIN, D. E. (1971) Depression: A Behavioral Formulation. *Archives of General Psychiatry* 24: 515–23.

LOGAN, W. P. D. and CUSHION, A. A. (1958) *Morbidity Statistics for General Practice* Vol. 1, General Register Office No. 14. London: HMSO.

MCKINLAY, J. (1972) Some Approaches and Problems in the Study of the Use of Services – An Overview. *Journal of Health and Social Behaviour* 13: 115.

MCMAHON, J. T. (1964) The Working Class Psychiatric Patient: A Clinical View. In F. Riessman, J. Cohen, and A. Pearl (eds.), *Mental Health of the Poor*. New York: The Free Press.

MACNAMARA, M. (1974) Talking with Patients, Some Problems met with by Medical Students. *British Journal of Medical Education* 8: 17.

MAGUIRE, G. PETER (1976) The Psychological Social Sequella of Mastectomy. In J. Howells (ed.), *Modern Perspectives in Psychiatric Aspects of Surgery*. New York: Brunner-Mazel.

———, CLARKE, D., and JOLLY, B. Unpublished.

———, JULIER, D. L., HAWTON, K. E. and BANCROFT, J. H. J. (1974) Psychiatric Morbidity and Referral on Two General Medical Wards. *British Medical Journal* i: 286.

——— and RUTTER, DEREK R. (1976a) History-taking for Medical Students: Deficiencies in Performance. *Lancet* ii: 556–58. See Reading 6.

——— (1976b) Training Medical Students to Communicate. In A. E. Bennett (ed.), *Communication between Doctors and Patients*. Oxford: Oxford University Press.

MAHLER, HALFDAN (1975) Health – A Demystification of Medical Technology. *Lancet* ii: 829–33, November 1. See Reading 30.

MANTEL, N. and HAENSZEL, W. (1959) Statistical Aspects of the Analysis of Data from Retrospective Studies of Disease. *Journal of the National Cancer Institute* 22: 719–48.

MARINKER, M. (1970) Truce. In Michael Balint, J. Hunt, D. Joyce, M. Marinker, and J. Woodcock (eds.), *Treatment or Diagnosis: A Study of Repeat Prescriptions in General Practice*. London: Tavistock Publications.

MARKS, R. V. (1967) Factors Involving Social and Demographic Characteristics: A Review of Empirical Findings. *Millbank Memorial Fund Quarterly* XLV(2) part 2: 41–8, April.

MAUKSCH, H. O. (1972) Ideology, Interaction and Patient Care in Hospitals. Paper presented at the Third International Conference on Social Science and Medicine, Elsinore, Denmark.

MAYER, JOHN E. and TIMMS, NOEL (1969) Clash in Perspective between Worker and Client. *Social Casework* 50: 32–40, January. See Reading 11.

——— (1970) *The Client Speaks: Working Class Impressions of Casework*. London: Routledge & Kegan Paul.

MECHANIC, D. (1962) The Concept of Illness Behaviour. *Journal of Chronic Diseases* **15**: 189.

MEIGS, J. W. (1961) Occupational Medicine. *New England Journal of Medicine* **264**: 861–67.

MERTON, R. K. (1957) *Social Theory and Social Structure*. New York: The Free Press.

MORRELL, D. C. (1972) Symptom Interpretation in General Practice. *Journal of the Royal College of General Practitioners* **22**: 297.

———, GAGE, H. G., and ROBINSON, N. R. (1970) Patterns of Demand in General Practice. *Journal of the Royal College of General Practitioners* **19**: 331.

NEYMAN, J. (1950) *First Course in Statistics and Probability*. New York: Holt.

NORMAN, J. C. (1969) Medicine in the Ghetto. *New England Journal of Medicine* **281**: 1271.

NOYCE, J., SNAITH, A. H., and TRICKEY, A. J. (1974) Regional Variations in the Allocation of Financial Resources to the Community Health Services. *Lancet* **i**: 554–57.

OVERALL, B. and ARONSON, H. (1964) Expectations of Psychotherapy in Patients of Lower Socioeconomic Class. *American Journal of Ortho-psychiatry* **33**: 421–30.

PARSONS, TALCOTT (1950) Illness and the Role of the Physician. *American Journal of Orthopsychiatry* **21**: 452–60.

——— (1951) *The Social System*. Glencoe, Illinois: The Free Press.

PAUL, B. D. and MILLER, W. B. (eds.) (1955) *Health, Culture and Community: Case Studies of Public Reactions to Health Programs*. New York: Russell Sage Foundation.

PEARSE, I. H. and CROCKER, L. H. (1954) *The Peckham Experiment*. London: Allen & Unwin.

PRUGH, D., STAUB, E., SANDS, R., KIRSCHBAUM, R., and LENIHAN, R. (1953) A Study of the Emotional Reactions of Children and Families to Hospitalization and Illness. *American Journal of Orthopsychiatry* **23**: 70–106.

QUERIDO, A. (1958) *Folia Psychiat. heerl.* **61**(220): 156. No. 2 Rumke Volume.

——— (1959) Forecast and Follow-up. *British Journal of Preventive and Social Medicine* **13**: 33–45. See Reading 19.

QUERIDO, A., VAN DER MEULEN, L. H. D., and WILLEMSE, W. J. Z. (1955) Inleiding tot een integrale geneeskunde. Leyden: Sterfert Kroese.

RADKE-YARROW, MARIAN, SCHWARTZ, CHARLOTTE GREEN, MURPHY, HARRIET, S., and DEASY, LEILA CALHOUN (1955) The Psychological Meaning of Mental Illness in the Family. *Journal of Social Issues* **11**: 12–24. See Reading 7.

RAHE, R. H., GUNDERSON, E., and RANSOM, J. A. (1970) Demographic and Psychosocial Factors in Acute Illness Reporting. *Journal of Chronic Diseases* **23**: 245.

REA, J. N. (1972) Personal Communication.

REIN, MARTIN (1969a) Social Class and the Utilization of Medical Care Services. *Journal of the American Hospital Association* **43**: 54.

————— (1969b) Social Class and the Health Service. *New Society* 14: 807.

RICHARDSON, S. A., DOHRENWEND, B. S., and KLEIN, D. (1965) *Interviewing: Its Forms and Findings*. New York: Basic Books.

RICHMOND, J. B. and WEISSMAN, H. A. (1955) Psychological Aspect of Management of Children with Malignant Diseases. *American Journal of Diseased Children* 89(42).

ROGHMANN, K. J. and HAGGERTY, R. J. (1972) The Diary as a Research Instrument in the Study of Health and Illness Behaviour. *Medical Care* 10(2): 143.

ROSENBERG, MORRIS (1963) Parental Interest and Children's Self-conceptions. *Sociometry* 26: 35–49.

————— (1968) *The Logic of Survey Analysis*. New York: Basic Books. See Reading 4.

ROSENGREN, WILLIAM R. and DEVAULT, SPENCER (1964) The Sociology of Time and Space in an Obstetrical Hospital. In Eliot Freidson (ed.), *The Hospital in Modern Society*. New York: The Free Press. See Reading 22.

ROSENMAN, RAY H., FRIEDMAN, MEYER, STRAUS, REUBEN, WURM, MOSES, KOSITCHEK, R., HAHN, W. and WERTHESSEN, N. T. (1964) A Predictive Study of Coronary Heart Disease: The Western Collaborative Group Study. *Journal of the American Medical Association* 189: 15–26.

—————, —————, STRAUS, REUBEN, JENKINS, RICHARD J., ZYANSKI, S.J., and WURM, MOSES (1970) Coronary Heart Disease in the Western Collaborative Group Study: A Follow-up Experience of 4½ Years, *Journal of Chronic Diseases* 23: 173–90.

—————, BRAND, RICHARD J., JENKINS, C. DAVID, FRIEDMAN, MEYER, STRAUS, REUBEN, and WURM, MOSES (1975) Coronary Heart Disease in the Western Collaborative Group Study: Final Follow-up Experience of 8½ Years. *Journal of the American Medical Association* 233: 872–77. See Reading 26.

ROYAL COLLEGE OF GENERAL PRACTITIONERS WORKING PARTY (1972) *The Future General Practitioner*. London: Royal College of General Practitioners.

RUTTER, DEREK R. and MAGUIRE, G. PETER (1976) History-taking for Medical Students II – Evaluation of a Training Programme. *Lancet* ii: 558.

RUTTER, MICHAEL L. and BROWN, GEORGE W. (1966) The Reliability and Validity of Measures of Family Life and Relationships in Families Containing a Psychiatric Patient. *Social Psychiatry* 1: 38.

SCHEFF, THOMAS J. (1963) Decision Rules, Types of Error and their Consequences. *Behavioural Science* 8: 97–107. See Reading 27.

————— (1964) Preferred Errors in Diagnosis. *Medical Care* 2: 166–72.

SCHMALE, A. H. JR (1958) Relationship of Separation and Depression to Disease 1. A Report on a Hospitalised Medical Population. *Psychosomatic Medicine* 20: 259.

SCHOFIELD, MICHAEL (1965) *The Sexual Behaviour of Young People*. London: Longmans.

SCOTT, R. and MCVIE, D. H. (1962) Doctor in the House: An Analysis of House Visits in General Practice. *Journal of the Royal College of General Practitioners* 5: 72.

SEEMAN, MELVIN (1959) On the Meaning of Alienation. *American Sociological Review* **24**: 783–91, December.

SELIGMAN, M. E. P. (1975) *Helplessness: On Depression, Development and Death*. San Francisco: Wilt Freeman.

SHERIF, M. and HOVLAND, C. I. (1961) *Social Judgement*. New Haven: Yale University Press.

SIEGEL, G. S. (1963) *Periodic Health Examinations – Abstracts from the Literature*. Public Health Service Publication No. 1010. Washington, DC: US Government Printing Service.

SKIPPER, JAMES K. and LEONARD, ROBERT C. (1968) Children, Stress, and Hospitalization. *Journal of Health and Social Behavior* **9**: 275–86. See Reading 21.

————, ————, and RHYMES, J. (1968) Child Hospitalization: An Experimental Study of Mothers' Stress, Adaptation and Satisfaction. *Medical Care* **6**: 496–506.

SMITH, T. (1967) Factors Involving Sociocultural Incongruity: A Review of Empirical Findings. *Millbank Memorial Fund Quarterly* **LXV(2)** part 2: 23–40.

STELLING, JOAN and BUCHER, RUE (1973) Vocabularies of Realism in Professional Socialization. *Social Science and Medicine* **7**: 661–75. See Reading 18.

STIMSON, GERRY and WEBB, BARBARA (1975) *Going to See the Doctor*. London: Routledge & Kegan Paul. See Reading 16.

SUCHMAN, EDWARD A. (1967) Appraisal with Implications for Theoretical Development of Some Epidemiological Work on Heart Disease. *Millbank Memorial Fund Quarterly* **XLV(2)** part 2: 109–113. See Reading 3.

SZASZ, THOMAS (1961) *The Myth of Mental Illness*. New York: Harper & Row.

TAPIA, F. (1972) Teaching Medical Interviewing: A Practical Technique. *British Journal of Medical Education* **6**: 133.

TIME MAGAZINE (1968) To Save the Heart; Diet by Decree?: January 10: 42.

TITMUSS, RICHARD M. (1968) *Commitment to Welfare*. London: Allen & Unwin.

TOWNSEND, PETER (1974) Inequality and the Health Service. *Lancet* **i**: 1179–190.

TUCKETT, DAVID A. (ed.) (1976) *An Introduction to Medical Sociology*. London: Tavistock Publications.

VAUGHN, CHRISTINE E. and LEFF, JULIAN P. (1976a) The Measurement of Expressed Emotion in the Families of Psychiatric Patients. *British Journal of Social and Clinical Psychology* **15**: 157–65. See Reading 2.

————, ————, (1976b) The Influence of Family and Social Factors on the Course of Psychiatric Illness: A Comparison of Schizophrenic and Depressed Neurotic Patients. *British Journal of Psychiatry* **129**: 125–37.

WADSWORTH, M. E. J., BUTTERFIELD, W. J. H., and BLANEY, R. (1971) *Health and Sickness: The Choice of Treatment*. London: Tavistock Publications.

WALLER, J. J. and MORRELL, D. C. (1972) Multidisciplinary Research in General Practice. Scientific Meeting of Staff of Academic Departments of General Practice, Cardiff, June. Unpublished.

WARREN, F. W. (1973) A Teacher Looks at Todd. *University of London Bulletin* No. 11, October.

WARREN, J. V. and WOLTER, JANET (1954) Symptoms and Diseases Induced by the Physician. *General Practitioner* 9: 77–84.

WEDGE, B. (1961) Psychiatry and International Affairs. *Science* 157: 281–85.

WEIJEL, J. H. and WILLEMSE, W. J. Z. (1955) *Mogelijkheden van integraal-geneeskundig werk in het ziekenhuis.* Amsterdam.

WHITE, K., ANDJELKOVIC, A., PEARSON, R. J. C., MABRY, J. H., ROSS, A. and SAGAN, O. K. (1967) International Comparisons of Medical Care Utilization. *New England Journal of Medicine* 277: 516–22.

WING, JOHN K. (1961) A simple and Reliable Sub-classification of Chronic Schizophrenia. *Journal of Mental Science* 107: 862.

———— (1970) A Standard Form of Psychiatric Present State Examination and a Method of Standardizing and Classification of Symptoms. In E. H. Hare and John K. Wing (eds.), *Psychiatric Epidemiology.* London: Oxford University Press.

————, BENNET, D. H., and DENHAM, J. (1964) The Industrial Rehabilitation of Long-stay Schizophrenic Patients. *Medical Research Council Memo* No. 42. London: HMSO.

————, BIRLEY, J. L. T., COOPER, J. E., GRAHAM, P., and ISAACS, A. D. (1967) Reliability of Procedure for Measuring and Classifying 'Present Psychiatric State'. *British Journal of Psychiatry* 113: 449–515.

———— and BROWN, GEORGE (1970) *Institutionalism and Schizophrenia: A Comparative Study of Three Mental Hospitals 1960–68.* Cambridge: Cambridge University Press. See Reading 23.

————, COOPER, J. E., and SARTORIUS, N. (1974) *The Measurement and Classification of Schizophrenic Symptoms: An Instruction Manual for the Present State Examination and CATEGO Programme.* London: Cambridge University Press.

———— and FREUDENBERG, R. K. (1961) The Response of Severely Ill Chronic Schizophrenic Patients to Social Stimulation. *American Journal of Psychiatry* 118: 311.

————, MONCK, E., BROWN, G. W., and CARSTAIRS, G. M. (1964) Morbidity in the Community of Schizophrenic Patients Discharged from London Mental Hospitals in 1959. *British Journal of Psychiatry* 110: 10.

WOOTTON, B. (1959) *Social Science and Social Pathology.* London: Allen & Unwin.

ZOLA, IRVING KENNETH (1972) Medicine as an Institution of Social Control. *Sociological Review* (new series) 20(4): 487–504. See Reading 28.

———— (1973) Pathways to the Doctor – From Person to Patient. *Social Science and Medicine* 7: 677–89. See Reading 14.

Indexes

Name index

Subject index